Healing Torah

Where healing, love and nature come together.

Oren Amber Ph.D.

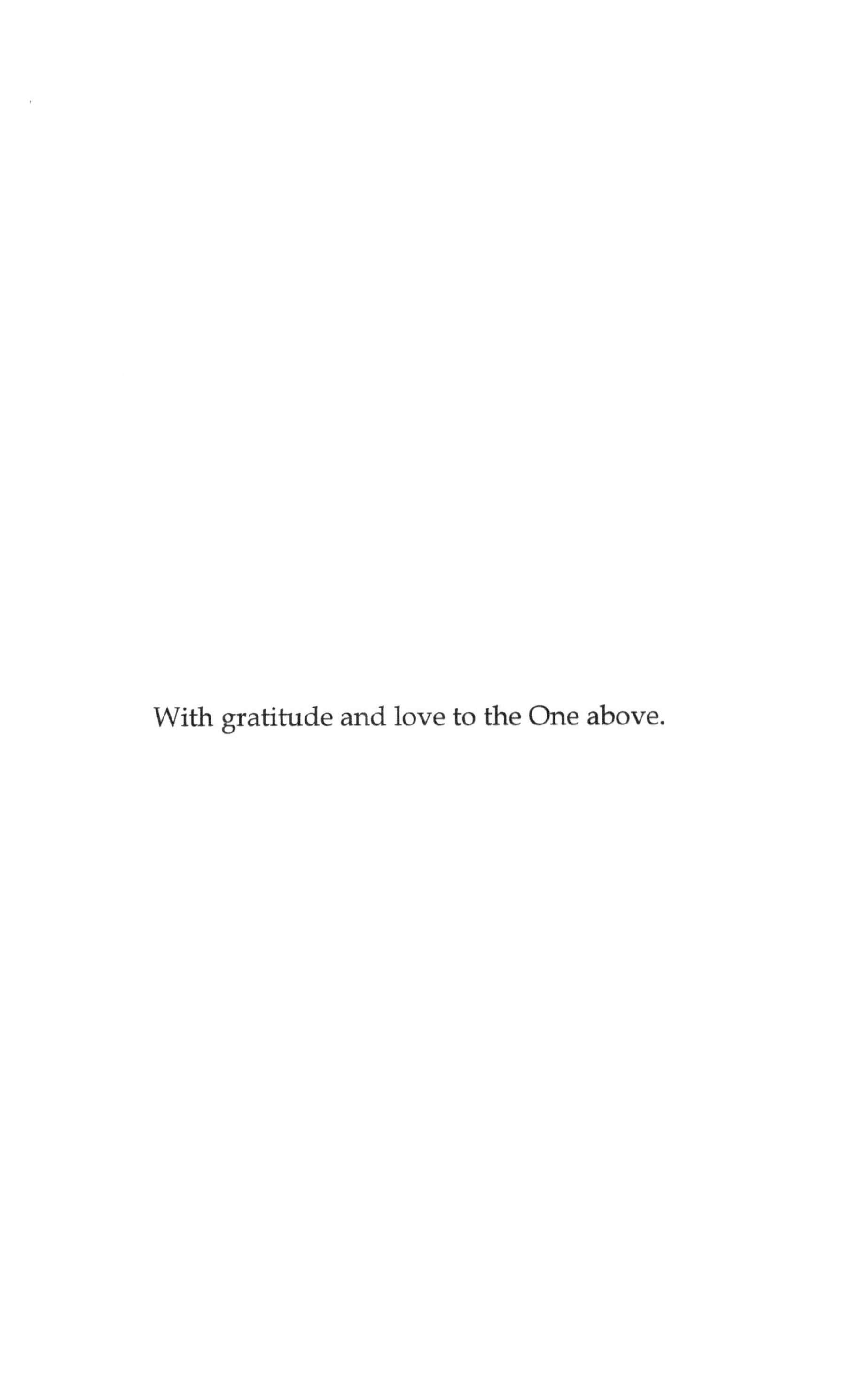

With gratitude and love to the One above.

By the stream, on its bank from either side, will grow
every tree for food; its leaf will not wither, neither will
its fruit end; month after month its fruits will ripen, for
its waters will emanate from the Sanctuary, and its
fruit shall be for food and its leaves for a cure.

Ezekiel 47:12

CONTENTS

Introduction

Thousands of years later the Torah is still teaching us, among much other wisdom, the essence of healing and blessed ways to live our life. It took me many years to understand the answer I got from a monk while trying to enter a monastery in Far East Asia, telling me "Go home to your religion. You have everything you need in it." Hopefully this book will help you, the truth seeker, to find your path.

"…May your heart keep My commandments; for they shall add length of days and years of life and peace to you…it shall be healing for your navel and marrow for your bones…Length of days is in its right hand; in its left hand are riches and honor. Its ways are ways of pleasantness, and all its paths are peace. It is a tree of life for those who grasp it, and those who draw near it are fortunate (Proverbs 3:1, 2, 8, 16, 17, 18).

Most of my life I was the active kind of guy. I was into

jogging, power walking, was the captain of a basketball team and even hiked the Himalayas. I majored in the health science field in college and worked as a caregiver, but it felt all the time that I was missing a big part of the puzzle. I remember once hearing that we have lost our sixth sense and if we are lucky, we can bring it back through fixing our eating habits, which will affect our connection to the Divine. It took me about 36 years of my life to understand and experience this. After all if we won't eat and drink, we will become souls again, which means that food is the major connector between physicality and spirituality.

So I decided to continue with the searching and to go and learn religious studies and live a religious lifestyle. I have to admit that it felt like a huge piece of the puzzle was found and I felt closer to Source. Still, on a physical level, I felt foggy, not so focused and drained. It felt like there was not enough light in my eyes. They were not as bright as I remembered them. I suddenly realized that I had gained weight and had a little belly. I decided to go for a checkup after about ten years of not seeing a doctor, as much as I remembered.

To my surprise a very slim, fit, tall grey-haired physician came into the room and pretty quickly raised his voice telling me, "Young man you are neglecting yourself. You have to start taking care of yourself. What about starting with losing some weight? You know you are overweight right?" I am quite a direct person myself but I was not used to having direct people around me. I felt that my eyes were getting wet and butterflies in my chest were trying to escape, but they didn't know the way out. I thanked him with a choked voice and went to the other room to take an EKG test. The nurse came in, looked at me for a second and said "I think I'll give you a few minutes to yourself. Call me when you're ready." The minute the door shut I started crying and crying and crying. I didn't know what had hit me. I think that it was the first time in a while that someone had told me the truth to my face, without fancy words or fake smiles, just straight to the point. I think that I was disappointed, embarrassed and hurt from myself: How did I get here? The one that never had to worry about weight, was always slim and fit, Mr. Young forever, Mr. healthy and spiritual.

I know you probably think what's the big deal, nothing happened. Well for me it was a big deal, because it was a sign of a wrong turn in my life. You see, I had worked in hospitals and taken care of enough patients to understand that we should not wait to get sick to see the stop sign in front of our eyes. We need to learn to be sensitive enough to see the warning lights and take a healthy turn. The problem was that I didn't know how and where to turn to. I was sitting in the clinic room by myself, wearing the patient coat this time, asking the One above with tears in my eyes to help me to see the way, to open my eyes and to give me the wisdom. After thinking for a while and trying to figure out where to start, I decided to start with the health food store down the road. I had been there before, but it was the first time that being there made me feel safe. I felt like I just wanted to move in. I think I must have spent at least two hours there, mostly in the reading corner. I felt a great thirst for information about a healthy lifestyle. Just like in my spiritual studies, the more I read the more I understood how much I didn't know or how much there is to learn. You see this kind of stuff they don't teach you in school. And when I say school I mean kindergarten, elementary school, junior high and college.

It's amazing that in an average of seventeen years of education nobody teaches you how to eat healthy, live healthy or lose weight. I remember buying a book with about 800 pages packed with information. My wife and I read it like a suspension novel. It felt like it was the beginning of a new piece of the puzzle, a new part of Godliness that was missing, another part of the quiet truth. From that point on, the health food store became my second home. It felt as if this store was like an angel that was sent from above to help us with the confusion on our planet. Organic fruits and vegetables, pure water and no entry for pesticides and preservatives felt like another right step to take. The next step was visiting the park. It's interesting how every change in our diet has an effect on us. I guess we all know the saying "we are what we eat" but it's different to see it happening in our life. I suddenly remembered the beautiful park next to my house. I had lived in that neighborhood for a couple of years and I think I had been to the park twice. It's funny how much easier it is to plan a vacation than to plan a visit to the park, which is usually free of charge and open 24/7. Anyway, it was a beautiful day and I got to power walk, stretch, watch the squirrels and even some rabbits, enjoy the amazing sun, which I had forgotten existed, and see and talk to other people who were practicing healthier habits. I got home a little sore and tanned and even a little smile started to show.

I started doing this about five days a week. I felt much better and much more positive. I even lost a few pounds, but then I realized that I wanted to lose more weight and I had no clue how to even start, since I had never had the need to lose weight. I understood that there are no short cuts. Everything we do has an effect on us, what we eat, what we don't eat, when we work out, when we sit on the couch, the decisions we make, even when we are just smiling to others.

Seeing these ideas in front of my eyes, I understood that I had to search more and try to create little healthy habits. After all it's all about the little details right?

After checking out some books I realized that like anything else there are many ways and several opinions for each way. The truth is that none of them seemed "healthy" enough to me and definitely not a way to follow for a long time or as a way of life. Just like many other times in my life the search, the time and the patience paid off. I felt blessed to find my new path. It felt like another big piece of the puzzle of life that I had been trying to put together was found.

If you are wondering about me and my puzzle and how I knew if it was the right piece or not, if it was a big piece or a small piece. All I can tell you is that the answers are all within us, but many times it takes time and tricks to get it out. When you find it, you feel that a great light was added to your soul. I guess you simply feel more complete. I hope it makes sense.

Anyway the basic idea of this radiant life style is to eat mostly fresh fruits and vegetables, nuts and seeds as organic, clean and close to creation as possible. Juices, smoothies, salads, soups, etc. Well, you are probably asking, "So what is there to eat?" There is plenty to eat! It just takes a little time to adjust, to look at the kitchen differently and to learn some new recipes like raw vegan pizza, pasta, couscous or crackers, etc. With a little creativity the sky is the limit. What's interesting is that after you become familiar with this way of eating, you realize how it's all in our heads. When you eat "couscous" without wheat, only using vegetables and it tastes the same if not better, you understand it's all in our heads. With the help of the One above and with this brilliant lifestyle I dropped 50 pounds in about 3 months and have succeeded in maintaining a healthy weight and lifestyle.

In this book I am sharing with you years of searching and precious information from my journey. I hope you will find this information helpful and interesting and that it will bring wellness, light and love to your life like it did to mine.

1
Genesis

"Bereishit bara Elokim…"

"At first the Creator created…" (Genesis 1:1).

Nothing that happens is a coincidence and definitely the fact that the Hebrew word for the Creator is "Boreh", for created "bara", for creation "briah" and for healthy "bria". There must be a reason why these four words have the same three root letters. In different words, in order to be "bari" - healthy, you need to strive to know and connect to the Creator - "Boreh" and that's done by knowing, appreciating and guarding the Creator's creation - "briah". It is also not a coincidence that the numerical value of one of the Hebrew Names of God "Elokim" has the same numerical value as the Hebrew word nature "HaTeva". This explains why some people interchange the terms "God" or "Creator" with the terms "Nature" or "Universe".

Within this book, whenever one of these terms is used,

the reference is to the Creator, an ungraspable force which was is and will always be.

The Rambam (Maimonides, 1135-1204) one of the greatest scholars and physicians said, "Since the body being healthy is of the ways of Hashem, for it is impossible to understand or know the knowledge of the Creator while unwell, therefore, one should keep away from things which destroy the body and accustom oneself to healthy and curing matters" (Hilchot Deot ch. 4). After writing Principles of Health in the "Book of Mada", the Rambam concludes that whoever will follow such a path is guaranteed not to become sick all his life but will leave this world at a ripe old age, without needing a doctor. His body will be whole and healthy for his entire life unless it was impaired from birth, he had been accustomed to bad habits from birth or if a plague, pestilence or drought occurred (Hilchot Deot ch. 4). Being healthy is our natural state and is the birthright of all creations. The wise ones will connect themselves to Source, learn the true teachings and spend their life trying to understand and practice this wisdom. Our conclusion is that in the beginning the Creator created a healthy creation. In Hebrew: "Haboreh bara briah bria". By connecting to the Creator, and following the rules of creation, we should live a long, happy and healthy life.

Three fundamental and eternal teachings can be found in the book of Genesis. First, "And God formed man of dust from the ground, and He breathed into his nostrils the soul of life, and man became a living soul" (Genesis 2:7). We can learn to respect and guard the soil that we came from and the air we breathe. Second, "God said behold, I have given to you all herbage yielding seed that is on the surface of the entire earth and every tree that has seed-yielding fruit; it shall be yours for food" (Genesis 1:29). We can learn that the ideal human diet is fresh fruits and vegetables, nuts and seeds. King Solomon, the wisest of all men says: "My fruit is better than gold, than fine gold and my produce than choice silver" (Proverbs 8:19). Thousands of years later, in apparently the largest nutritional research conducted by Cornell University, Oxford University and the Chinese Academy of Preventative Medicine, they reached a similar conclusion (The China Study, 2006). It's unbelievable that we need a whole book to explain a very straight forward verse, but I guess that's how "sophisticated" we have become.

Third, "Now God took the man, and He placed him in the Garden of Eden to work it and to guard it" (Genesis 2:15). We can learn that the initial purpose that we the humans were put here for was to work and to guard the land. It's not a coincidence that two out of three Pilgrimage festivals are based on farming: the festival of harvesting – Shavuot and the festival of gathering the harvest – Sukkot. It's definitely not a coincidence that the acronym LOVE can stand for Live Organic Vegan Edibles. When you eat Godliness, you are filled with Godliness and love.

Love is a foundation of the world. The world was created with love and kindness and by us respecting and loving the Creator and the creations; we make this world a "Garden of Eden" and a heavenly place to live. Loving the Creator: "And you shall love your God, with all your heart and with all your soul, and with all your means" (Deuteronomy 6:5). Loving the creation: "In the beginning God created the heavens and the earth" (Genesis 1:1). When you love the Creator, you love the creations. Loving each other: "You will neither take revenge from nor bear a grudge…you will love your neighbor as yourself. I am God" (Leviticus 19:18). Loving animals: "If you see your enemy's donkey lying under its burden would you refrain from helping him? You will surely help along with him" (Exodus 23:5). Loving plants: "When you besiege a city for many days to wage war against it to capture it, you shall not destroy its trees by wielding an ax against them, for you may eat from them, but you shall not cut them down. Is the tree of the field a man, to go into the siege before you?" (Deuteronomy 20:19). Loving the earth and the air: "And God formed man of dust from the ground, and breathed into his nostrils the soul of life, and man became a living soul" (Genesis 2:7). "Do not draw near here. Take your shoes off your feet, because the place upon which you stand is holy soil" (Exodus 3:5).

"How precious is Your kindness, O God! Mankind takes refuge in the shelter of your wings. They will be sated from the abundance of Your house; and from the stream of Your delights You give them to drink. For with You is the source of life; by your light may we see light" (Psalm 36, 8-10). When we connect to Source we understand that there is a perfectly accurate order and rhythm to creation. Every little thing has a job; every little thing has a purpose. By truly internalizing this concept and practicing it, we keep the balance. When we try to outsmart these ways and look for shortcuts i.e. genetically engineering our food and spraying and poisoning our soil, fruits and vegetables, etc., this is when the imbalance begins and "genetically engineered" chaos in the shape of unwellnesses and other catastrophes might come to visit.

"My soul, bless Hashem! Hashem my God, You are greatly exalted; You have garbed Yourself with majesty and splendor. You enwrap with light as with a garment; You spread the heavens as a curtain. He roofs His heavens with water; He makes the clouds His chariot, He moves on the wings of the wind. He makes the winds His messengers, the blazing fire His servants.

He established the earth on its foundations that it shall never falter. The depths covered it as a garment; the waters stood above the mountains. At Your warning they fled; at the sound of Your thunder they rushed away. They ascended mountains, they flowed down valleys, to the place which You have assigned for them. You set a boundary which they may not cross, so that they should not return to engulf the earth. He sends forth springs into streams; they flow between the mountains. They give drink to all the beasts of the field; the wild animals quench their thirst. The birds of the heavens dwell beside them; they raise their voice from among the foliage. He irrigates the mountains from His clouds above; the earth is satiated from the fruit of Your works. He makes grass grow for the cattle, and vegetation requiring the labor of man to bring forth food from the earth; and wine that gladdens man's heart, oil that makes the face shine, and bread that sustains man's heart. The trees of Hashem drink their fill, the cedars of Lebanon which He planted, wherein birds build their nests; the stork has her home in the cypress. The high mountains are for the wild goats; the rocks are a refuge for the rabbits. He made the moon to calculate the festivals; the sun knows its time of setting. You bring on darkness and it is night, when all the beasts of the forest creep forth. The young lions roar for prey, and seek their food from God. When the sun rises, they return and lie down in their dens. Then man goes out to his work, to his labor until evening.

How manifold are Your works, O Hashem! You have made them all with wisdom; the earth is full of Your possessions. This sea, vast and wide, where there are countless creeping creatures, living things small and great; there ships travel, there is the whale that You created to frolic therein. They all look expectantly to You to give them their food at the proper time. When You give it to them, they gather it; when You open

Your hand, they are satiated with goodness..." (Psalm 104). As we said before, at first the creation was perfectly healthy, organized and in balance. It didn't take too long to become greedy and to eat from the "forbidden" tree – the tree of knowledge, trying to outsmart the advice of the Creator. Then we tried to reach Heaven with the tower of Babel. Then came the idea of bowing down to money and possessions in the shape of a golden calf, etc. In short, we chose the "smart and sophisticated" way and guess what, Mr. Chaos and his friends came to visit. It got to the point that we need to pay a fortune of money and go to special stores in order to be able to bite into a fruit that was not sprayed with sophisticated poison that can hardly be washed off, or was changed genetically and is no longer the "child" of another fruit and the list goes on.

The Creator gave the soil the power of growth so that when we plant a seed it would grow and we could be nourished from it and live a long and healthy life. Before the flood, people lived to be almost 1000 years old. On a common sense level this should be enough in order to treat the land properly but for whatever the reason some decided that there are no rules or rhythm to this creation, so they started poisoning it with pesticides, herbicides, fungicides, radiation whatever works so maybe they'll be capable of making a few more pennies. Remembering "Hashem God formed the man of dust from the soil and He blew into his nostrils the soul of life and the man became a living being" (Genesis 2:7) might help us to respect the earth and the air which the Creator set as a must for our existence. We all need to follow the true laws of the universe. It is for our own good. Here are some examples: A Sabbatical year for the land once every seven years: "But in the seventh year, the land shall have a complete rest a Sabbath to Hashem; you shall not sow your field, nor shall you prune your vineyard. You shall not reap the after growth of your harvest, and you shall not pick the grapes you had set aside, it shall be a year of rest for the land" (Leviticus 25:4-5).

The jubilee year as a year of rest for the land: "It is a Jubilee year for you, the fiftieth year, you shall not sow, you shall not harvest its after growth and you shall not pick what was set aside of it for yourself…You shall perform My decrees, and observe My ordinances and perform them; then you shall dwell securely in the land. The land will give its fruit and you will eat your fill; you will dwell securely upon it…I will ordain My blessing for you in the sixth year and it will yield a crop sufficient for the three year period" (Leviticus 25:11, 18-21). The obligation to preserve fruit trees: "When you besiege a city for many days to wage war against it to capture it, you shall not destroy its trees by wielding an ax against them, for you may eat from them, but you shall not cut them down. Is the tree of the field a man, to go into the siege before you?" (Deuteronomy 20:19). To breed animals and sow seeds according to their kind: "You shall observe My laws: You shall not crossbreed your animals with different species. You shall not sow your field with a mixture of seeds…" (Leviticus 19:19). When we should eat fruit from a new tree: "When you come to the Land and you plant any food tree, you shall surely block its fruit; it shall be blocked from you for three years, not to be eaten. And in the fourth year, all its fruit shall be holy, a praise to Hashem. And in the fifth year, you may eat its fruit; to increase its produce for you. I am Hashem, your God" (Leviticus 19:23-25).

How to harvest: "When you reap the harvest of your Land, you shall not completely remove the corner of your field during your harvesting, and you shall not gather up the gleanings of your harvest. You shall leave these for the poor person and for the stranger. I am Hashem, your God" (Leviticus 23:22).

So what can we do? Some say we should just go to nature and ask the Creator to show us the way. "A psalm by David. Hashem is my shepherd, I shall lack nothing. He lays me down in green pastures; He leads me beside still waters. He revives my soul; He directs me in paths of righteousness for the sake of His Name" (Psalm 23). Others learn from books or from each other, "Ben Zoma said: Who is wise? He who learns from every person as it says: From all those who have taught me I have gained wisdom" (Psalm 119, Avot 4:1).

"The foundation of all foundations and the pillar of wisdom is to know that there is a Primary Being who brought into being all existence. All the beings of the heavens, the earth, and what is between them came into existence only from the truth of His being. If one would imagine that none of the entities aside from Him exist, He alone would continue to exist, and their nullification would not nullify His existence, because all the entities require Him and He, blessed be He, does not require them nor any one of them. Therefore, the truth of His being does not resemble the truth of any of their beings" (Rambam Yesodei haTorah 1:1-3).

There are many ways to find answers but the "master key" is to try to connect to the original plan and the way things were meant to be, to make our home and environment the "Garden of Eden". To work towards having a pure heart, body, mind and soul, pure water, pure air, pure nutrition, etc.

It is interesting that one of the calculations of the numerical value of the Hebrew word "eitz" (tree) is 7 (70 + 90 = 160. 1+6+0=7). This reflects 7 lessons we can learn from a tree: Just like the air in the forest is usually pure and clean, "A person should always try to live in a place where the air is pure and clean..." (Kitzur Shulchan Aruch 32:25). Just like trees get their water through their roots, their filtration system from deep in the ground where the water is usually pure, a person should drink only pure water: "Concerning drink, water is the most natural drink for man, and healthy for the body, as long as it is pure and clear, it leads to preserving the body fluids and speeds up the evacuation of waste products..." (Kitzur Shulchan Aruch 32:17).

Just like trees must have sunlight in order to grow, a person should get enough sunlight to allow the body to produce sufficient amounts of vitamin D, which is necessary for growth.

Just like there are plants which go to sleep at night by closing their petals and wake up by opening them at sunrise, a person should make sure to get enough sleep each night in order to get up with sunrise: "The day and the night together are twenty four hours. It is sufficient for a person to sleep a third of the total, which is eight hours. They should be at the end of the night in order to have from the beginning of his sleep until sunrise eight hours, so he should be out of bed before sunrise" (Rambam Hilchot Deot, ch. 4).

"Now the sun was ready to set, and a deep sleep fell upon Avram" (Genesis 15:12). Just like the tree stretches in the wind with its branches and leaves, a person should stretch and exercise every day, especially before eating: "It is an important principle of medicine that before eating one should walk or exercise until the body has warmed up and then eat. As it says, "By the sweat of your brow, you should eat your bread (Genesis 3:19) and not eat the bread of idleness (Proverbs 31:27)..." (Kitzur Shulchan Aruch 32:6).

Just like the trees are silent, never angry, grow towards Heaven, bend their "head" in humility when the wind blows and "clap" their leaves thanking their Creator, a person should "...increase in silence and should speak only when he has a wise thing to say or for the sake of his needs..." (Rambam Hilchot Deot, ch. 2:4). Rabbi Shimon the son of Rabban Gamliel said, "All my days I grew up among the Sages and did not find anything better for one's person than silence..." (Avot 1:17). Rabbi Akiva said, "...a fence for wisdom is silence" (Avot 3:13). A person shouldn't be angry and should be humble: "And when you will be saved from anger the attribute of humility will come upon your heart an attribute which is the best of all good attributes..." (Igeret haRamban).

A person should give thanks to the Creator: "Give thanks to Hashem for He is good, for His kindness is forever" (Psalms 136:1). Just like trees share their fruits and allow us to use their logs to build and heat our homes, a person should be busy with doing kindness (gemilut hasadim) and be willing to sacrifice for others when needed (mesiroot nefesh), without expecting something in return. Other than these amazing free gifts that trees give us and the great lessons we can learn from them, they also protect us from air pollution and environmental toxins. In the same way we should protect our planet, our home and our bodies.

I believe that this beautiful creation we all live in has everything we need in it, which brings me to believe that if we are lacking something it has to be somewhere around us.

2
Sophisticated Toxins

While many of us are familiar with air and water pollution sources like cars, public transport, aircraft, nuclear, oil, coal, gas, oil refinery, ethanol biorefinery, liquefied natural gas, trash, biomass, meat production, tire incinerating, landfill, landfill gas burners and sewage incinerators as opposed to green non polluting energy sources such as solar, wind and hydro and while it is possible to find information about the air quality in your city and county by visiting different websites such as: the American Lung Association State of the Air, AirNow for the air quality index (AQI) and Energy Justice Map (Network), not too many are familiar with indoor pollution which is much harder to detect.

The healthier I ate and the more I changed my lifestyle, the more sensitive I became to my own feelings, to others and to the environment. With the sensitivity of my palate I revealed a completely new and beautiful world. Not only did the food taste different, the sounds around me got clearer. The noise of traffic became louder, while the sound of the quiet and the birds sounded much more rich and beautiful to the level of feeling that I could almost understand what they were saying.

Another sense that seemed to get stronger and clearer was my sense of smell. It was like I gained a pair of turbo nostrils. Many times I could smell very gentle aromas from the other side of the house. It's funny but I started to feel like I became the bionic man. Suddenly I couldn't take the smell of the plastic shower curtain, the scented soaps and some fabrics I was surrounded by. I realized that there is an underground world of toxins in my own home. I feel that because of lack of attention or knowledge and sometimes just a matter of price or convenience, toxins find easy access into our homes, offices, etc. While some of the more obvious ones are in cigarette smoke, some cleaning products, pesticides, aerosol sprays etc., some of the more sophisticated ones are in synthetic fabrics and fabric dyes, different kinds of plastics, paints, cosmetic products, drinking and shower water etc. So what can we do? Here are a few tips to try out: Living in an area with clean air away from traffic, power plants, etc., using kitchen and shower water filters, using 100% cotton linen and towels, wearing natural fabrics, filling our home with plants to purify the air, getting rid of plastic or aluminum as much as possible and using wood, glass, ceramics or stainless steel instead, removing cleaning or cosmetics products which contain toxic chemicals and avoiding the use of toxic paint.

If it feels overwhelming remember that just by being aware, we are half way there. Finding out about the high amount of toxins which were in my basic daily hygiene products like toothpaste, deodorant, hand cream, etc., I felt a need to look for alternatives. It made no sense to me to slowly poison myself, even though it was in small amounts. My poor armpits, which for the best of my knowledge were created to get toxins out of my body, should not be blocked at all, especially not with sticky stuff which contains aluminum and or other interesting ingredients. I found out that what creates the sweaty smell is actually bacteria not the sweat itself, which makes a lot of sense.

Well, guess what did the deodorant trick? Believe it or not, baking soda. All I did was simply pour the baking soda into a shaker with wide enough holes, or simply took it straight out of the package and put a little under my arms after the shower, while my armpits were still damp. You don't need to put very much. Surprisingly enough it lasted and it worked. For me it works longer than regular deodorant and I don't think we need to mention the money I save.

For hand lotion I use a combination of olive oil and coconut oil. The ratio is 1 part olive oil to 2 parts coconut oil. It depends on the consistency you like. For a firmer consistency, add more coconut oil. In order to melt the coconut oil, I place it into a small dry bowl and put this bowl into a small tub of hot water until it becomes fluid. Then I mix it with the olive oil. For fragrance I add some lemon juice or cinnamon. Then I mix it, pour it into a container, preferably a glass one, and put it into the fridge until it sets.

As far as shampoo, I know that some people use a combination of apple cider vinegar and lemon juice. It's also possible to find clean products at the health food store. But still, don't forget to check the ingredients on the label, no matter where you buy it, especially for ingredients such as SLS or sodium lauryl sulfate, which is used as a foaming agent.

Another one I struggled with was cleaning the hot water urn or the electric kettle. It made no sense to me to use strong chemical solutions. The best cleaning solution that I came up with was using citric acid. Boiling 1 to 2 tablespoons of citric acid in the amount of water that covers the residue did the job. I reboiled the solution or added more citric acid depending on how severe the build-up was. It was interesting to see that when using reverse osmosis filtered water there was no mineral residue or build-up at all.

3
EMF

"I saw and behold there was a stormy wind coming from the north, a great cloud with igniting fire and illumination surrounding it and from it like Electricity coMing out of the Fire" (Ezekiel 1:4). "…there is illumination to the fire and from the fire lightening comes out" (Ezekiel 1:13). EMF is a subject that I tried to learn a lot about and I asked many questions, but there weren't too many answers. It seems that nobody knows exactly how EMFs operate and the exact damage they can cause. One thing that everyone agreed is that the safest is when appliances are unplugged. EMF stands for Electro-Magnetic Field. Magnetic fields are measured using milli-Gauss (mG). Apparently the field is strongest near the source and becomes weaker the further away you move from it. These fields are able to affect particles from far away. This is how wireless technology is possible. According to the Swedish government the established safety limit for exposure to ELF (Extremely Low Frequency) magnetic field is 2.5 mG, and VLF (Very Low Frequency) magnetic fields is only 0.25 mG. It could mean that consistent exposure exceeding the standard, might be a risk for developing health problems which can range from headaches, fatigue, and dizziness to skin rashes, miscarriage, leukemia, etc. The problem is it seems that the rest of the world is going through the same process that it went through with the tobacco industry.

Even though many people suspected and believed in the danger of cigarette smoking and the connection between smoking and different deadly unwellnesses it seems like it took forever to become an official and recognized danger. I was shocked to find old commercials on YouTube of doctors advertising cigarettes. Today, while smoking is not allowed in public places, cell phones, laptops, computer screens, and other interesting electronic devices surround us almost everywhere we go. Not to mention the new babysitter of the generation – computer games on cell phones played by infants who are still growing and developing. Did you know that a hair dryer, which people hold only a few inches from their brain, can give off an astounding few hundred mG! While like we mentioned above, according to the Swedish government, 2.5 mG should be the limit.

So what can we do with this information? The best advice I can give from my personal experience is simply to buy an EMF detector on Amazon or Ebay. It might not be 100% accurate but it can do the job of this extra sense we are missing and give you a good idea of how far to stay away from appliances in order to be under 2.5 mG or as low as possible. It can also help in deciding if you want these devices in your environment at all and can help to detect hidden cables and or wires in the walls.

Additional practical and easy advice is to unplug unneeded appliances, keep a distance from electric devices, become friendly with your EMF detector and take it with you to places where you and your family spend your time, for example, work, school, the car, etc. You will probably be surprised by your detective work as was I. Another good idea is to look around your house and to see how close or how far you are from electric wires outside the house, which might also be high EMF sources. Although this meter can give you a good idea of what's going on, you might need a professional assessment. In that case remember to ask for an official report and advice of how to take the matter further if needed. If this all sounds a little way out there or like a Ghostbusters story, I witnessed a close relative revealing, with a $10 EMF detector, an illegal electric cable that was located under her office. An official report that was ordered later showed a reading of around 16 mG which is over 6 times the Swedish recommendation. Many times using corded instead of cordless appliances might be safer. Try to have the places where you spend most of your day as far as possible from EMF sources.

4
GMO, Kilayim
& Organic

"…you shall not mate your animal into another species, you shall not plant your field with mixed seed…" (Leviticus 19:19).

"Hashem created the world with certain distinct species and His wisdom decreed that these species remain intact and unchanged. For man to take upon himself to change the order of creation suggests a lack of faith in Hashem's plan. Moreover, each species on earth is directed by a Heavenly force so that each species found on earth represents profound spiritual forces. To tamper with them is to cause harm that man living on earth cannot begin to understand…Animals shall not give birth to a species that is not their own, since the resulting animals will not be able to multiply. The same thing applies to plants. Also mixing seeds is forbidden since they will be changed in their nature and shape, while nourishing from each other. Each seed will be as if it is made of two species..." (Ramban Leviticus 19:19). Genetically modified foods are foods that come from genetically modified organisms which have been altered using genetic engineering methods. These foods were first sold to the public in the early 1990s. There are many concerns about the safety of GM foods and their potential harming effect on our health and the environment.

Potential health risks associated with genetically modified foods have been found in various studies (AAEM 2009). These include accelerated aging, immune problems, infertility, faulty insulin regulation, and changes in major organs and the gastrointestinal system. There is also concern about the impact that genetically modified crops may have on the environment. It may take years to see the real impact of these foods on people, animals and the environment. After all GMOs are human-made mutations of the creation. Some countries do not allow GMOs to be used in food production at all, while others use a staggering amount (over 90%) of GMO in commonly used produce like sugar beets, cotton, soy, and corn. Non GMO labeled products do not contain GMOs but may still be grown using synthetic fertilizers, pesticides, herbicides, etc.

Organic produce is grown without the use of synthetic fertilizers, pesticides, herbicides, the neurotoxin hexane, genetically modified organisms, sewage sludge, antibiotics, or ionizing radiation. It has been proven to be more nutritious and to contain up to 100 times less pesticide residue when compared to non-organic produce. The dangers of consuming synthetic pesticides are well known. Pesticides have been linked to, Alzheimer's Disease, ADHD, birth defects and cancer and could potentially harm the nervous, reproductive and endocrine systems. Washington State University quotes Pullman Wash. which found that organic foods and crops have many advantages over their conventional counterparts, including more antioxidants and fewer, less frequent pesticide residues.

So what can you do? If you have a backyard, you can try to grow your own produce using organic, non GMO seeds. Another option is indoor gardening. Try to buy only organic foods if possible, or look out for the organic and non GMO label on produce and products. At the very least become familiar with the list of foods that are more prone to be highly sprayed such as strawberries, spinach and apples and those that are likely to be genetically engineered like corn, soy and sugar beet. You can try to avoid these foods if they are not organic or non GMO. In general it is always a good idea to read labels. It is wise to be aware of what is entering our system and what is in our surroundings i.e. the ingredients in the food we eat, the ingredients that we don't understand or can't pronounce, the ingredients in vaccinations, the ingredients used at the dentist's office, the ingredients in the clothes we wear, the ingredients in our cosmetics and personal hygiene products and if we are not happy with these, what are our alternatives? Reading the label is one of the only ways to know what you are putting into your body.

So what about all the toxins that are already in our system? A healthy body removes toxins naturally. However due to the excessive amount of toxins that we are exposed to in our days, the body can get overloaded and may need some help. It is possible to get a general picture of the amount of heavy metal and chemical toxicity in the body by doing a hair analysis.

There are different opinions of how to remove these from the body. One idea is to use chelation therapy that binds the toxins in the bloodstream by circulating a chelating solution. Examples of natural chelators which you can include in your diet are cilantro, garlic, onion, and selenium. Chelating agents can be taken orally and are available in over-the-counter formulas or they can be administered in intravenous solutions under the supervision of a physician.

The chelators pull out toxic metals and other harmful substances which impair body function and help the body remove these toxins via the kidneys. Eating a high fiber diet and using coffee or water enemas may also be helpful in flushing out these toxins. Some say a clean food-based multivitamin supplement should be consumed during the process. The idea is to take in as few toxins as possible and to remove as many toxins from the body as we can. Generally speaking in all aspects of our life we should try to remove the negative and bring in the positive as much as possible. Hashem created the world with infinite wisdom. We see it time and time again. It's amazing how not keeping one little verse as mentioned above can cause so much chaos and unwellnesses and take things out of balance in ways that are extremely difficult, if not impossible to reverse.

5
A Fundamental Idea In Health

The acid level in our body is measured by the pH level. It ranges from 0-14, where 7 is neutral, 14 is the most alkaline and 0 is the most acidic. While toxins, stress, parasites, high amounts of acid-forming food such as white sugar, most of the grains and beans, meat, fats, animal protein, pasteurized dairy, very few fruits for example tomatoes and very few nuts like peanuts, can tilt the body towards the acidic side, high amounts of most fresh fruits and vegetables, especially fresh and organic green-leafy vegetables can tilt the body towards the alkaline side. Green-leafy vegetables are blood purifiers, antibacterial, antioxidant, liver detoxifiers, energy boosters and rich in enzymes as well. It doesn't mean not to ever eat a tomato but understand that eating tomato soup and other acid-forming foods everyday probably would tilt the system towards the acidic side.

So why is this information so important? Well, on a simple level an alkaline body will be at less risk of unwellness if at all. Or in other words theoretically we shouldn't become unwell if we keep our body slightly alkaline. Diseases apparently need an acidic environment to survive. Research has proven that disease cannot survive in an alkaline state, and that bacteria, viruses, mold, yeast, fungus, candida and cancer cells thrive in an acidic, low oxygen, low pH environment. Most pathogens and cancers cannot survive in an oxygen-rich, alkaline environment. One explanation is that the more alkaline the blood, the more oxygen it should be able to absorb. That's why physical exercise, which increases the oxygen supply to our body, is extremely important as well. Just think about the word "acid" compared to the word "greens". Which would you prefer to have in your body?

So how can you know how alkaline or acidic you are? All you need to do is buy litmus paper or pH test paper and test your urine. It can be measured by testing blood or saliva as well. Some say to test once a day. The best is first thing in the morning before eating, or one hour after. Others suggest testing every time you urinate within 24 hours, to write down the reading and then to average the results. My understanding is that it depends on what you are trying to achieve. If you just want to know, what your pH level is in general, then you can test once first thing in the morning. If you want a more accurate pH reading, try the 24-hour average. If you are not happy with your pH level and you are trying to correct it, then test for several days, once a day, every time you urinate, or go for a blood test, depending on the accuracy you are after. Remember that the results are affected by what you ate the day before. If you feel that you would like to be more on the alkaline side, try to incorporate more alkaline-forming foods.

6
Water

This upgraded lifestyle kept bringing me back to that lesson in elementary school about photosynthesis. I am sure that you all remember that one. If a plant needs sun, water and good soil to grow then what about us? I realized that I was hardly drinking water. Not a good habit, considering that we can't live more than three days without it. Our bodies are about 60% water. Drinking water can be very helpful with skin rejuvenation, toxin elimination, relieving constipation, losing weight, improving blood circulation and increasing energy and alertness. So, the first question is: How much water should I drink? Well, the truth is that we are all different and that there are many factors involved i.e. the climate, the season, the temperature, our body weight, our lifestyle, our age, our eating habits.

So I think that's why it's hard to find one absolute answer. I have heard different opinions: 33 fluid ounces (about a liter or 4 cups) a day, 66 fluid ounces or until the color of the urine is clear. Another opinion is to watch out not to get the kidneys to work too hard and if the color is clear, it means that we are drinking too much. The reason behind this is that too much water makes it harder for the system to remove waste. According to this opinion, clear urine means that water left the body, but not so much waste. That's why we should look for clear light yellowish colored urine as an indicator for drinking the right amount of water.

Another idea is that if you are in-tune with your body, it should be enough to drink when you are thirsty, otherwise you should try to drink three to four cups a day. These are some different opinions and suggestions. Try and see which works best for you.

Another question I had was what kind of water I should drink? Looking around and seeing all the different bottled water companies and all the different water filtration systems was a little hint about the tap water quality problem our precious planet is having. It looks like we have polluted most of the water sources available to us. Toxins find their way into our water from many sources like acid rain, sewage, industrial overflow, pipe leakage, chlorine and the list goes on. A good way to measure water quality is to use a TDS (Total Dissolved Solids) meter that can be purchased online for less than $10.

There are many different types of water i.e. tap, bottled, de-ionized or de-mineralized, ground, spring, mineral, sparkling, carbon-filtered, distilled, reverse osmosis, etc. The general idea is to drink and cook in pure, clean water. I am the type of person that likes to see what the products that I am taking into my body went through. That's why I felt safer to use a home water filtration system.

After extensive research, I narrowed down my choices to three: steam-distilled: the water is heated to boiling point and the condensed steam is captured, reverse osmosis: the water is forced through a semi-permeable membrane which filters contaminants, and activated carbon-water: the water is filtered through a carbon trap which absorbs the contaminants. Considering factors like the price, the number of contaminants being filtered, user friendliness and taste, I chose the reverse osmosis for drinking and food preparation. A few years later I still feel it was a great choice.

7

Liquid Sunshine

One of the essentials in today's world is the daily Green Juice - a chlorophyll rich drink. A popular nick name for chlorophyll is "liquid sunshine". It is the light of the sun that is absorbed in the green pigment of living plants and is packed with a range of powerful nutrients including vitamins A, C, E, K, beta-carotene, antioxidants, magnesium, iron, potassium, calcium, and essential fatty acids Usually the greener and darker the surface of the plant, the richer it is in chlorophyll with chlorella being said to have the highest concentration. Chlorophyll is like the blood of the plants. Its molecular structure is very similar to the structure of the hemoglobin in our blood. The difference is that hemoglobin is built around iron, whereas chlorophyll is built around magnesium. Chlorophyll can act as a blood purifier, is anti bacterial, an antioxidant, a liver detoxifier, an energy booster and is enzyme-rich. It might be helpful in regulating blood sugar levels, high blood pressure, some skin problems, anemia and improving digestion. Leafy greens are rich in amino acids and packed with vitamins and minerals. Another important value of greens is that they help to keep our body alkaline. The idea of green juice is to use many kinds of green leafy vegetables like spinach, celery, lettuce, parsley, alfalfa sprouts, etc. You can mix them altogether if you like. Then it's up to you. Some say not to mix fruits and vegetables, in which case you would add carrots for some sweetness. Others say we should only mix apples with the greens and the vegetables. If you can't get used to the taste, it is suggested to have your greens with whatever works for you. Some add bananas or dates to mask the flavor of the greens. Eventually your taste buds will get used to the yummy flavor of the "magical greens".

You can juice your greens using a cold press juicer or simply using a blender. Pretty much any blender can work. If using a blender, first add some pure, clean water that will at least cover the blades. Then add your greens with whatever your choice of fruits or vegetables and blend. The idea is to create as little foam as possible, since foam means oxygenation and the more oxygenation, the more loss of nutritional value. Then pass the juice through a piece of cloth or a nut-milk bag to separate the pulp from the juice. Drinking the juice without pulp ensures easier and faster absorption of the vitamins and minerals.

Three advantages of juicing over eating fruits and vegetables: First, it is much easier to drink the amount of a packed blender than to chew it. Imagine how long it would take to eat the amount of greens that can fit into a blender. Second, the body uses much less energy when drinking than when chewing. The less energy you use the more you have. Third, to the best of my knowledge, juice gets absorbed into our bodies much faster than food does, to the extent that some say it is absorbed into our blood stream before it even gets to the large intestine. Whoever is looking for the highest quality juice, with the least oxygenation and the highest nutritional value, will probably use a twin-gear, low-speed juicer. A popular brand is the "Green Star" juicer. In case you are making wheat grass juice, use only a juicer, which is designed for juicing wheatgrass. Not separating the pulp properly might be dangerous as grass cannot be digested and might stick to the intestinal walls. Green juices are rich in minerals, enzymes and vitamins and are absorbed almost entirely in our digestive system. It is important to consume a variety of green vegetables since each has its own unique nutrient profile. It is best to make them with organic vegetables and to drink them right away. Other than having healthy eating habits, juices are great to add to your daily menu, especially due to the nutrient depletion of the soil in our generation and the need to consume larger amounts of greens and vegetables in order to supply the needed amount of nutrients.

8
Seven Super Foods & Healing Plants

"For Hashem your God is bringing you to a good land, a land with brooks of water, fountains and depths that emerge in valleys and mountains. A land of wheat and barley, vines and figs and pomegranates, a land of oil producing olives and honey…And you will eat and be sated, and you shall bless Hashem, your God, for the good land He has given you a land in which you will eat bread without scarcity, you will lack nothing in it, a land whose stones are iron, and out of whose mountains you will hew copper" (Deuteronomy 8:7-10).

"If only My people would listen to Me, if Israel would go in My ways…He would feed him with the fat of wheat and I would satisfy you with honey from a rock" (Psalm 81:14, 17).

WHEAT GERM

Rich in vitamin E, and contains most of the B vitamins,

magnesium, calcium, phosphorus and some trace elements. Wheat germ can help to decrease free radicals in the body, prevent disease, boost immunity, maintain healthy weight, control cholesterol levels and keep the heart and cardiovascular systems healthy.

WHEAT GRASS JUICE

A nutritionally complete food, and contains 17 amino acids, is extremely rich in protein, rich in minerals, contains vitamin A, B-complex, C, E and K as well as trace elements and enzymes. Wheat grass juice is antibacterial and can be an effective healer, can help to slow down the aging process, help to keep the hair from graying, remove heavy metals, clear up congestion, purify the liver, improve blood sugar levels, help to prevent tooth decay, help to treat blood disorders and neutralize toxins. High in chlorophyll, wheatgrass can be very effective in treating anemia and in treating many other disorders. Used topically it can be beneficial in the treatment of various skin diseases.

It has been said that 1 ounce of wheatgrass juice is equivalent nutritionally to 2 pounds of vegetables.

BARLEY AND BARLEY GRASS JUICE

Rich in calcium, iron, chlorophyll, flavonoids, vitamin B12 vitamin C and contains all the essential amino acids, many minerals and enzymes. Barley grass juice can heal the stomach, duodenal and colon disorders and can be effective as an anti-inflammatory.

GRAPES AND GRAPE JUICE

Rich in phytonutrients, mainly phenols, and polyphenols, and contain vitamins A, K, C, and vitamin B6. They are also contain thiamine, niacin, riboflavin, and folate, potassium, magnesium, calcium, phosphorus, and sodium. Grapes can treat constipation, indigestion, fatigue, macular degeneration, kidney disorders, and prevent cataracts. Grapes can help to keep the body hydrated, and also contain dietary fiber, carbohydrates, antioxidants, and some protein. Flavonoids in grapes can slow down aging and help to reduce the damage caused by free radicals.

GRAPE SEED EXTRACT AND OPCS

Rich in flavonoids with antioxidant capabilities. Oligomeric Proanthocyanidin known as OPCs can protect the brain and spinal nerves from free radical damage, protect the liver from damage, strengthen and repair connective tissue, support the immune system, slow down aging and can moderate allergic and inflammatory responses by reducing histamine production.

FIGS

"The eyes of both of them were opened, and they knew they were naked, and they sewed fig leaves and made themselves girdles" (Genesis 3:7).

While the first garment in the garden of Eden was fig leaves, which made some people refer to the fig tree as the tree of knowledge, it is interesting to find that fig tree leaf extract may have anti-wrinkle capabilities for the skin, which is our natural garment.

Rich in calcium, fiber and antioxidants and contain manganese, magnesium, copper, potassium, vitamin K, and vitamin B6. Figs can act as an antibacterial and antifungal agent, regulate blood sugar levels, prevent macular degeneration, treat anemia, liver disease, paralysis, ulcers, skin diseases, gastrointestinal tract and urinary tract infections, aid in weight loss, inhibit kidney and liver problems, cancer and high blood pressure, and protect the heart.

POMEGRANATE

Rich in antioxidants, vitamins C, E, K, folate, and potassium. Pomegranates are antibacterial and antiviral and can help to remove free radicals, reduce inflammation, protect cells from damage, stop the growth of prostate cancer cells, protect memory, improve learning, slow down the progress of Alzheimer disease, improve digestion, help lower systolic blood pressure, protect the arteries and heart, prevent illness and fight off infection, aid in fertility, reduce inflammation in the gut helping with inflammatory bowel diseases such as Chron's disease and ulcerative colitis, help decrease insulin resistance and lower blood sugar, help reduce soreness and improve strength recovery following exercise.

OLIVE, OLIVE OIL AND OLIVE LEAVES

Rich in Oleuropein. Antioxidant, antiviral, anti-inflammatory, antibacterial and can help to protect against infection, be useful in treating pneumonia, skin disorders, sore throat, sinusitis, provide immune and cardiovascular support and increase energy.

HONEY

"So Israel, their father, said to them, "If so, then do this: take some of the choice products of the land in your vessels, and take down to the man as a gift, a little balm and a little honey, wax and lotus, pistachios and almonds" (Genesis 43:11). The common opinion is that the Torah is referring to date honey.

DATES

Contain fiber, potassium, calcium, magnesium, iron, phosphorus, zinc, sodium, thiamin, vitamins A, K, riboflavin, folate, and niacin. Dates can help with weight loss, digestive health, reduce heart disease risk, relieve constipation, support regular bowel movements, help with impotence, promote heart health, relieve diarrhea, reduce blood pressure, help with iron-deficiency anemia, aid in hemorrhoid prevention, promote respiratory health, help with chronic conditions such as arthritis, reduce colitis risk and prevent colon cancer.

EZEKIEL BREAD RECIPE

"And you, take yourself wheat and barley, and beans

and lentils, and millet and spelt. You shall place them in one vessel, and prepare them for yourself as bread the number of days that you lie on your side, three hundred and ninety days you shall eat it" (Ezekiel 4:9). Even though the connotation of this bread was not the most positive one, Ezekiel bread has become a very popular health bread today.

OTHER HEALING HERBS AND PLANTS

"And Hashem said to Moses: "Take for yourself aromatics, balsam sap, onycha and galbanum, aromatics and pure frankincense; they shall be of equal weight" (Exodus 30:34).

BALSAM SAP

Topical applications: can be used as a painkiller, antiseptic, healing ointment for wounds such as cuts, abrasions, burns, sores, and chapped areas. As a warm tea mixed with water or eaten directly: can help with bronchitis, rheumatism or inflammation, cough, sore throats, cancer, dysentery, inflammation of the mucus membranes, scurvy, heart ailments, colds, flu, earache, urogenital ailments such as gonorrhea and vaginal infections, pain in the muscles and joints, and ulcers. As an inhalant: for headaches.

ONYCHA

As an essential oil: anti-inflammatory, expectorant, antioxidant, antiseptic, contracts body tissues, deodorant, cleanser for cuts and wounds, diuretic, and sedative.

GALBANUM
As a gum-like material (resin) from the roots and trunk of a tree and can be applied directly to the skin for wounds. In food and beverages, galbanum oil and resin are used as flavoring.

FRANKINCENSE
Most known for incense, frankincense was used during ceremonial offerings. It is an anti-inflammatory agent, antidepressant, sedative and analgesic. Frankincense oil can also used to improve anxiety.

"Hashem spoke to Moses, saying: "And you, take for yourself spices of the finest sort: of pure myrrh five hundred shekel weights; of fragrant cinnamon half of it two hundred and fifty shekel weights; of fragrant cane two hundred and fifty shekel weights, and of cassia five hundred shekel weights according to the holy shekel, and one hin of olive oil" (Exodus 30:22-24).

MYRRH
Myrrh was used as an ingredient in the anointing oil used in the Tabernacle. In the Roman world, it was considered a natural remedy for almost every human affliction from earaches to hemorrhoids. It is anti-parasitic, antibacterial and antifungal.

CINNAMON

Once considered more precious than gold. The bark, where the oil comes from, was collected for anointing oil, as well as perfume. Cinnamon can be used to lower blood glucose levels, is antifungal, can be used to treat athlete's foot and yeast infections and can help to calm the stomach.

CASSIA

"Vedan and Javan gave spun silk into your treasure houses, iron wrought into ingots, cassia and calamus was in your stores" (Ezekiel 27:19). Cassia oil was popularly used as anointing oil during Biblical times and has aromatic properties similar to cinnamon. It is used in natural hair care, coloring and conditioning. Anti-diarrhea, stimulant, anti-rheumatic, antiviral, circulatory, antidepressant, antimicrobial, anti-arthritic, can reduce vomiting and nausea, decrease milk secretion, relieve skin irritations, relieve flatulence, invoke menstruation and reduce fever.

BALM

"And they sat down to eat a meal, and they lifted their eyes and saw, and behold, a caravan of Ishmaelites was coming from Gilead, and their camels were carrying spices, balm, and lotus, going to take down to Egypt" (Genesis 37:25). Balm or balsam refers to an extremely fragrant resinous substance extracted from a plant. It was considered extremely valuable. The balm or balsam of Gilead was named for the region of Gilead where it was made and this balm was used medicinally. It can be used as herbal ointments and oils to improve the health of the skin, reduce inflammation, speed wound healing, prevent infection, protect dental health, protect the respiratory system, and soothe hemorrhoids.

BITTER HERBS

"…they should eat…bitter herbs" (Exodus 12:8). Bitter herbs is a term used for foods such as endive, tansy, horseradish, horehound, parsley and coriander seeds. Bitter herbs were mostly used for food in the Torah. In fact, the children of Israel were commanded to eat bitter herbs on Passover. Bitter herbs can help with urinary tract infections, fluid retention, achy joints, kidney stones, gout and digestive troubles.

CUMIN

"Is it not so? When he smoothes its surface, he scatters the black cumin and casts the cumin, and he places the prominent wheat, and the barley for a sign, and the spelt on its border" (Isaiah 28:25). Cumin seeds were dried and used to flavor food. It can be used in fighting diabetes and has anticancer properties.

HYSSOP

"Purify me with a hyssop, and I will become pure; wash me, and I will become whiter than snow" (Psalm

51:9). Hyssop is a sweet smelling plant from the mint family and was used in ceremonial rituals. Hyssop can help with hyperglycemia, in tea and tincture form and can be used as an expectorant to improve respiratory related problems such as asthma, coughs and bronchitis. Warm hyssop tea or hyssop tincture diluted in warm water can be used as a gargling liquid for sore throats.

"Spikenard and saffron, calamus and cinnamon, with all frankincense trees, myrrh and aloes, with all the chief spices" (Song of Songs 4:14).

SPIKENARD

The oil stimulates the immune system, is anti-fungal, antibacterial, anti-inflammatory, relaxes the body and mind and can be used to treat stress, infections, digestive problems, and insomnia. It can also be used as a sedative, deodorant, uterine substance, and laxative.

SAFFRON

The most expensive spice in the world today was also very precious during ancient times. Due to its distinct yellow color, saffron was used for flavoring and to make dyes as well. In the past, people used saffron to treat stomach upsets, smallpox and bubonic plague. Saffron can produce a feeling of fullness for mildly overweight individuals, has cancer-inhibiting properties (specifically for breast cancer), and can have anti-depressant effects.

CALAMUS

The root can be used for gastrointestinal problems including ulcers, intestinal gas, inflammation of the stomach lining, loss of appetite and upset stomach.

FLAX

"Though the flax and the barley have been broken, for the barley is in the ear, and the flax is in the stalk" (Exodus 9:31). Flax contains omega-3 essential fatty acids which are known as "good" fats and are believed to have heart-healthy effects. Each tablespoon of ground flaxseed contains about 1.8 grams of plant omega-3s. Flaxseed contains 75 to 800 times more lignans than other plant foods.Lignans have both plant estrogen and antioxidant qualities. Flax can be used in helping improve cardiovascular health, cholesterol, digestion, skin, and hormone balance.

CUMIN

"Is it not so? When he smoothes its surface, he scatters the black cumin and casts the cumin, and he places the prominent wheat, and the barley for a sign, and the spelt on its border" (Isaiah 28:25). Rich in iron. Cumin has antiviral, antibacterial properties and contains an anticancer phytochemical. It can be used to treat respiratory disorders, aid digestion, stimulate acid secreting glands, bile and enzymes, boost the immune system, promote skin health, treat insomnia and prevent diabetes.

"We remember the fish that we ate in Egypt free of charge, the cucumbers, the watermelons, the leeks, the onions, and the garlic" (Numbers 11:5).

ONION
Contains phytochemicals, vitamin C and chromium. Onion can improve immunity, regulate blood sugar, reduce inflammation, heal infections, scavenge free radicals and reduce gastric ulcers.

GARLIC
In many cultures garlic has been used for thousands of years as both food and medicine. It contains calcium, folate, iron, magnesium, manganese, phosphorus, potassium, selenium, zinc, vitamins B1, 2, 3 and C. Garlic can boost the immune system, detoxify the body and protect against infection, enhance immune function, help prevent heart disease, help with hypertension, improve circulation, help with high cholesterol by lowering high lipid levels, stabilize blood sugar levels,

aid with arteriosclerosis, arthritis, asthma, colds and flu, digestive problems, heart disorders, insomnia, liver disease, sinusitis, ulcers, yeast infection and may help guard against cancer formation in the body.

Again we see the eternal wisdom of the Torah and how important it is to contemplate each word and not just take it at face value. While over 3000 years ago wheat and barley were mentioned as supreme foods, today wheatgrass and barley grass juices are being researched all over the world for their healing potential and are being used medicinally to treat terminal unwellnesses. The same applies to grapes with their bioflavonoids and treating heart conditions, honey, pomegranates, etc. Over 800 years ago the Rambam (Maimonides) wrote medical books with hundreds of healing plants. It feels like there will probably be more and more discoveries in the future about how these amazing foods that were specifically mentioned assist the body to do what it was created to do and heal itself.

9

Aromatherapy

"…how much better is your love than wine and the fragrance of your oils than all spices!" (Song of Songs 4:10). Fragrances and essential oils had an extremely important place in spiritual ceremonies. Twice daily every morning and evening, a mixture of spices were burnt on top of a golden alter. This alter was situated the closest to the holiest place in the Tabernacle, where the Ten Commandments were kept. Only once a year on the Day of Atonement fiery coals together with finely ground incense were taken into the Holy of Holies so that the cloud of incense would blanket the Ark cover. Only the priests were allowed to enter the place where they offered the incense and only certain people were allowed to prepare it. It was used in ceremonies in very accurate measures. A mistake in the measurement or ingredients would disqualify the incense from being offered. Moreover, the rest of the people were not permitted to copy the recipe and if someone did, they would be severely disciplined. Only the priests were allowed to partake in this sacred daily ceremony. Research is uncovering the properties and potential health benefits of aromatic spices which were used so many years ago. Today they can be used in the form of aromatherapy, which uses plant based materials and aromatic plant oils, including essential oils, to improve psychological or physical well-being. Aromatherapy utilizes naturally extracted aromatic essences from plants harmonizing, balancing and promoting the health of body, mind and spirit. It is said to affect through two basic mechanisms. One is the influence of aroma on the brain. The other is the direct pharmacological effects of the essential oils. Some of the potential benefits include pain and anxiety reduction, enhancement of energy and short-term memory, relaxation, hair loss prevention, reduction of eczema-induced itching, etc. Blends of therapeutic essential oils can be used in topical application, massage, inhalation or water immersion. Following are some ancient fragrances that were used thousands of years ago in the times of Moses and King Solomon: "…the fragrance of your garments is like the fragrance of Lebanon (Cedar)" (Song of Songs 4:11).

CEDARWOOD ESSENTIAL OIL

Mental focus, balancing and relaxing.

Cedarwood can help to heal wounds, help with dandruff, fight spasms, contract the tissues, gums, muscles, skin and blood vessels, increase urination, remove water, toxins, fat and salt from the body, help with coughs and colds, regulate menstrual cycles, kill insects, reduce inflammation and nervous disturbances and inhibit infections and fungal growth.

"Hashem spoke to Moses, saying: "And you, take for yourself spices of the finest sort: of pure myrrh five hundred of fragrant cinnamon half of it two hundred and fifty of fragrant cane two hundred and fifty and of cassia five hundred according to the holy shekel, and one hin of olive oil. You shall make this into an oil of holy anointment, a perfumed compound according to the art of a perfumer; it shall be an oil of holy anointment. And you shall anoint with it the Tent of Meeting and the Ark of Testimony, the table and all its implements, the menorah and its implements, the altar of incense, the altar of the burnt offering and all its implements, the washstand and its base. And you shall sanctify them so that they become a holy of holies; whatever touches them shall become holy" (Exodus 30:22-29).

MYRRH ESSENTIAL OIL
Confidence, strength and healing.
Myrrh has been used to restrain microbial growth, reduce hemorrhage and tighten gums and muscles. It is used to stop fungal growth, alleviate coughs and colds, reduce excess gas and stimulate discharges and systems. It can relieve phlegm, promotes sweating, is

good for stomach health, protects from infection, helps heal wounds quickly, improves circulation, boosts protection against diseases, boosts health and immunity, protects from rheumatism and arthritis, while also reducing spasms and sedating inflammation.

CINNAMON LEAF ESSENTIAL OIL
Can help in stopping diarrhea, hemorrhage and is a parasiticide.

CINNAMON ESSENTIAL OIL
Immune support. It is frequently used for blood impurity, blood circulation issues, respiratory problems, infections, wound healing, pain relief, birth control, menstruation problems, skin infections, breastfeeding, diabetes, heart disorders, colon cancer, indigestion, as a relief for bad breath and as a brain tonic.

CASSIA ESSENTIAL OIL
Cassia has been used to stop diarrhea, fight depression and uplift mood. It can reduce milk flow, inhibit microbial growth, stop vomiting, tighten gums and muscles, treat rheumatism and arthritis, and help stop hair loss. It is also thought to fight viral infections, reduce hemorrhaging, improve blood and lymphatic circulation, remove excess gas, relieve obstructed menstruation, and reduce fever.

"I am a rose of Sharon, a rose of the valleys" (Song of Songs 2:1).

ROSE ESSENTIAL OIL

Rose oil promotes a calm mood and fights harmful organisms. It contains tocopherol (vitamin E), carotene, and high levels of phenolic compound and can make the skin more permeable so it is often added to skin care products. It has been used to fight depression and uplift mood, protect wounds against developing sepsis, relieve spasms, fight viral infections, soothe inflammation due to fever, tighten gums and muscles, enhance libido and cure sexual disorders, and stop hemorrhaging. It also heals scars, opens up obstructed menses, inhibits bacterial growth, cures constipation and nervous disorders, promotes discharges and secretions, stops hemorrhaging, purifies the blood, boosts liver health, and is good for uterine and stomach health.

"And they sat down to eat a meal, and they lifted their eyes and saw, and behold, a caravan of Ishmaelites was coming from Gilead, and their camels were carrying spices, balm, and lotus, going to take down to Egypt" (Genesis 37:25).

The common name 'balm' is actually thought to be an abbreviation of Balsam (from Balsam of Gilead), the sweet smelling and mysterious 'chief of oils' and that lemon balm is related to the balm mentioned in the verse.

BALM OF GILEAD

It is used as an anti-inflammatory and diuretic.   Balm of Gilead promotes skin health, soothes the stomach and is beneficial for the immune system.

LEMON BALM ESSENTIAL OIL

Elevation of spirit and confidence.

Lemon balm is used to reduce the feeling of depression, open blocked menses, reduce spasms, help with nervous disorders, reduce inflammation, and is good for the stomach. It also removes gas, increases perspiration and removes toxins, inhibits bacteria, reduces fever, boosts the immune system and lowers blood pressure.

WHITE LOTUS ABSOLUTE OIL

Relaxant, aromatic and sedative.

PINK LOTUS ABSOLUTE OIL

Tonic, cardiac, lowers blood pressure and promotes digestion.

"Spikenard and saffron, calamus and cinnamon, with all frankincense trees, myrrh and aloes, with all the chief spices" (Song of Songs 4:14).

"While the king was still at his table, my spikenard gave forth its fragrance (Song of Songs 1:12).

SPIKENARD ESSENTIAL OIL

Spikenard has been used to eliminate body odor, inhibit bacterial and fungal growth, soothe inflammation and nervous disorders, clear the bowels, and restore uterine health.

SAFFRON ESSENTIAL OIL
Cheerfulness and wisdom.
Saffron can be used to treat light to moderate depression. It can be used to treat acne due to its anti-bacterial qualities.

CALAMUS ESSENTIAL OIL
Calamus essential oil can be used to treat rheumatism and arthritis, inhibits microbial growth, relaxes spasm, is good for the brain and memory, relieves nervous disorders, induces sleep and increases blood and lymph circulation.

FRANKINCENSE ESSENTIAL OIL
Peaceful, calm and comforting.
Frankincense essential oil protects wounds from becoming septic, induces contractions in gums, muscles, and blood vessels, heals scars, fights infections, removes excess gas, keeps cells healthy and promotes their regeneration, soothes anxiety and inflammation, increases urination, promotes digestion, regulates menstrual cycles, cures coughs and colds, and ensures good uterine health.

"Take for yourself aromatics, balsam sap, onycha and galbanum, aromatics and pure frankincense; they shall be of equal weight. And you shall make it into incense, a compound according to the art of the perfumer, well blended, pure, holy. And you shall crush some of it very finely, and you shall set some of it before the testimony in the Tent of Meeting, where I will arrange meetings with you; it shall be to you a holy of holies. And the incense that you make, you shall not make for yourselves according to its formula; it shall be holy to you for Hashem" (Exodus 30:34-37).

GALBANUM ESSENTIAL OIL

Galbanum has been used to treat rheumatism and arthritis, relax spasms, remove toxins, speed up the healing of wounds, clear scars and spots, improve skin health, clear congestion, increase blood and lymph circulation, ease breathing, eliminates parasites and kill and repel insects.

ONYCHA ESSENTIAL OIL

Onycha Essential Oil is an anti-inflammatory, expectorant, deodorant, antioxidant, antiseptic, diuretic, and sedative. It is used as an antiseptic and to clean cuts and wounds.

"Purify me with a hyssop, and I will become pure; wash me, and I will become whiter than snow" (Psalm 51:7).

HYSSOP ESSENTIAL OIL

Hormonal balance and calm breathing.

Hyssop can be used to reduce spasms, eliminate excess gas, tighten gums, muscles, skin and blood vessels, increase urination, heal scars and after-marks, reduce stress on the nervous system, promote digestion, increase blood pressure, decrease phlegm and coughs, regulate menstruation, promote sweating and reduce fevers.

"Your arid fields are as a pomegranate orchard with sweet fruit, henna and spikenard" (Song of Songs 4:13).

POMEGRANATE SEED ESSENTIAL OIL
Pomegranate seed oil contains punicic acid, an omega 5 fatty acid, which has strong anti-inflammatory properties. It can also provide protection against sun damage and keep the skin from ageing.

HENNA ESSENTIAL OIL
Calms the mind, body and soul, detoxifies and cools the body. Henna nourishes the hair and can prevent graying hair, dandruff and hair loss.

"...the fragrance of your countenance like apples" (Song of Songs 7:9).

APPLE SEED ESSENTIAL OIL
Rich in fatty acids which play an important role in the functioning of the body and enhance the appearance of the skin.

While in the past it looks like aromatherapy was practiced by using coals or applying carrier oils, especially olive oil, today there are many ways it can be administered like: aroma lamps or diffusers, carrier oils like sweet almond oil, essential oils, herbal distillates or hydrosols (by-products of the distillation process such as rosewater, lemon balm and chamomile) and vaporizers. Nowadays we see more and more awareness and appreciation for the magical gifts of nature and for the use of plants in the shape of aromatherapy, essential oils and oils in general for cosmetics, massage, healing and spiritual purposes.

10
Animal Products & The Environment

The original human diet: "And God said, "Behold, I have given you every seed bearing herb, which is upon the surface of the entire earth, and every tree that has seed bearing fruit; it will be yours for food" (Genesis 1:29). The Torah reminds us to be kind to animals: "If you see your enemy's donkey lying under its burden would you refrain from helping him? You shall surely help along with him" (Exodus 23:5). The Creator's response to animal sacrifice: "And Noah built an altar to Hashem, and he took of all the clean animals and of all the clean fowl and brought up burnt offerings on the altar. And Hashem smelled the aroma, and Hashem said to Himself, "I will no longer curse the earth because of man, for the imagination of man's heart is evil from his youth, and I will no longer smite all living things as I have done" (Genesis 8:20). The Creator's response to craving meat: "But the multitude among them began to have strong cravings. Then even the children of Israel once again began to cry, and they said, "Who will feed us meat?" (Numbers 11:4).

"…A wind went forth from Hashem and swept quails from the sea and spread them over the camp about one day's journey this way and one day's journey that way, around the camp, about two cubits above the ground.

The people rose up all that day and all night and the next day and gathered the quails. The one who gathered the least collected ten heaps. They spread them around the camp in piles. The meat was still between their teeth; it was not yet finished, and the anger of Hashem flared against the people, and Hashem struck the people with a very mighty blow.

He named that place Kivroth Hata'avah (Graves of Lowly Desires), for there they buried the people who craved" (Numbers 11:31-34). The reward for the correct path will be finest wheat and honey: "If only My people would listen to Me, if Israel would only walk in My ways, then I would quickly subdue their enemies, and turn My hand against their oppressors. Those who hate Hashem would shrivel before Him, and the time shall be forever. I would feed him with the finest of wheat and sate you with honey from the rock" (Psalms 81:14-17).

It feels like we have two brains; one in our head and one in our stomach. In order to have clarity, we need to clean our thoughts and our stomach. That is why it is so important to think positive thoughts, to eat the minimum needed and provide the stomach with healthy food.

The smart diet: "So Daniel said to the steward whom the chief officer had assigned to Daniel, Hananiah, Mishael and Azariah, "Please test your servants for ten days, and let them give us of the pulse and we will eat, and give us water and we will drink. Then let our appearance and the appearance of the youths who eat the king's food be seen by you, and act toward your servants in accordance with what you see." He heeded them in this matter, and tested them for ten days. At the end of ten days their appearance seemed better and they were of healthier flesh than the youths eating the king's food. Thereafter the steward would take away their food and their drinking-wine and give them pulse. As for these youths, the four of them, God gave them learning and skill in every script and wisdom; and Daniel understood every kind of vision and dreams. At the end of the years after which the king had said to bring them, the chief officer brought them before Nebuchadnezzar. The king spoke with them, and there was not found among them all anyone like Daniel, Hananiah, Mishael and Azariah; so they stood and served before the king.

In every matter of the art of reasoning that the king asked of them, he found them ten times better than the necromancers and astrologers that were in his entire kingdom" (Daniel 1:11-20). In times of wisdom, if lions will eat straw, what will man eat?! "And a shoot shall spring forth from the stem of Jesse, and a twig shall sprout from his roots. And the spirit of Hashem shall rest upon him, a spirit of wisdom and understanding, a spirit of counsel and strength, a spirit of knowledge and fear of Hashem. And he will be imbued with a spirit of fear of Hashem and will not need to judge by what his eyes see, nor decide by what his ears hear. And he will judge the poor justly, and decide with fairness for the humble of the earth, and he will strike the earth with the rod of his mouth and with the breath of his lips he will put the wicked to death. And righteousness will be the girdle of his loins, and faith the girdle of his waist. And a wolf will live with a lamb, and a leopard will lie with a kid; and a calf and a lion cub and a fatling together, and a small child will lead them. And a cow and a bear will graze together, their children will lie; and a lion, like cattle, will eat straw. And an infant will play by a viper's hole and a newly weaned child will stretch his hand toward an adder's lair. They will neither harm nor destroy on all My holy mountain, for the earth will be full of knowledge of Hashem as water covers the sea bed" (Isaiah 11:1-9). Respecting the creation is respecting the Creator: "…his mercy should extend to all creatures, neither destroying nor despising any of them. For the Supernal Wisdom is extended to all created things, inanimate, plants, animals and humans. This is the reason we were warned about not respecting foods. In this way man's pity should be extended to all the works of the Blessed One just as the Supernal Wisdom despises no created thing for they are all created from that source, as it is written: "In wisdom You have made them" (Psalms 104:24). In this way he should not treat any created thing without respect, for they were all created in Wisdom. He should not uproot anything which grows, unless it is necessary, nor kill any living thing unless it is necessary..." (Tomer Devora, end of ch. 3 by Rabbi Moshe Cordovero, master kabbalist, Israel, 1522-1570). "...honor all creatures, in which he recognizes the exalted nature of the Creator Who in wisdom created man. And so it was with all creatures, that the wisdom of the Creator is in them. He should see for himself that they are therefore to be honored exceedingly for the Creator of all, the most exalted Wise One has busied Himself with creating them and if man despises them, he touches upon the honor of their Creator, God forbid.

This can be compared to a wise jeweler who made a vessel with great wisdom and showed it to men, one of whom disrespects and speaks lightly of it. How angry that sage would be for by despising the work of his hands his wisdom is despised. And so it is in the eyes of the Holy One, Blessed is He, if any one of His creatures is despised. It is therefore written: "How manifold are Your works, Hashem..." (Psalms 104:24) not "how great", but "rabu", from the expression "rav beito" (Ester 1:8) namely, very important. "You have made them all in wisdom" (Psalms 104:24) and because Your wisdom is attached to your works, they are important and great. It is fitting that man see in them wisdom not cause for them to be despised" (Tomer Devora ch. 2). "Besides the cruelty of killing animals, which teaches a bad habit to the person…to shed innocent blood, eating some meat will bring thickness, turbidity and impurity to the soul…" (Sefer HaIkarim by Rabbi Yosef Albo, Spain, 1380-1444).

"…Without any sensitivity of justice and ethics that a person with the weakness of limitless self love approaches the poor cow and the mute ewe and takes from this one her milk and from the other her wool…There is no ethical problem if the wool is taken from the sheep at a time when the taking of the wool will lessen the burden of its owner or at least will not cause it sorrow or damage. But it's indecent when he takes it for his pleasure while the real natural owner, the actual sheep needs it. Then it is fitting, according to common sense, to recognize it as official theft which comes only from the advantage of the tough over the weak…"

"And the same idea applies to the milk that is being milked…There is connection between taking the milk from the animal and taking its life and its flesh from it. Meaning at a time and in a way that causes it sorrow and withholds the natural goodness and benefits which befit it."

"According to the complete view, which is full of the mercy of Hashem and His goodness for all His creations - a person will recognize the idea of milk existing in the breasts of the mother animal, not in order for he who has the power to exploit it for himself, but in order for the mother to breastfeed her tender child, her baby goat, that she loves, from the milk of her own breasts. This baby goat also deserves to have the pleasure of experiencing the love of its mother's breast in accordance with its character and nature. And the hardness of the human heart, which comes from its materialistic and moral weakness, has changed and twisted these straight and honest values. This baby goat would not be able, because of the low values of man, to enjoy the love of its mother and to rejoice as well in the ray of life. But it will be slaughtered and become food for the gluttonous stomach of man and for his low spirit which says: "Eat meat"…"

"No! The destiny of the baby goat is not necessarily to be food for your sharp teeth…and the milk in any case was not made to be a spice for you to fulfill your lowly desire…"

"You will know in time that the life of the living was not created for your gluttonous stomach and milk's main purpose is to be the nutrition for whomever nature came to feed. Just like the milk of your mother's breasts was a safe haven for you while you were breastfed…"(Tlalei Orot by Rabbi Avraham Yitzhak haCohen Kook, Latvia, 1865-1935). "In the future to come the level of animals will be as the level of man today, as a result of the elevation of the spiritual worlds" (Shaar haMitzvot, Parshat Ekev by Rabbi

Chaim Vital, Italy, 1543-1620, kabbalist and leading student of the Arizal). There is more and more research detailing the devastating effects on health as a result of consuming animal products. One of the most influential studies is "The China Study" conducted by Cornell University, Oxford University and the Chinese Academy of Preventative Medicine. Named "the Epidemiology Grand Prix" by the New York Times, it involved 6500 participants and is the most conclusive nutritional research ever conducted. The study concluded that the consumption of animal products dramatically increases the risk of obesity and many chronic diseases such as heart disease, cancer and diabetes. The environmental impact of meat production is tremendous. It uses vast amounts of land, water, and other resources to grow grains and other plants to feed animals which are then used for food. It would be much more environmentally efficient to feed people directly with plants.

As people's appetite for meat increases, countries all over the world are bulldozing land to make room for animals and the crops needed to feed them. From ancient pine forests in China to tropical rain forests in Brazil, entire ecosystems are being destroyed to sustain humans' addiction to meat.

Many times factory animal farming creates abusive conditions for animals as it strives to produce as quickly and cheaply as possible and in the smallest amount of space. The animals are kept in small cages, where they are often unable to turn around and are deprived of movement so that all their energy will go towards gaining weight and producing products for human consumption in the least amount of time. They are given drugs that fatten them more quickly, and they are genetically manipulated to grow faster or produce much more than they would or can naturally. Especially when we know the advantages of eating green on all levels physical, spiritual, environmental, how does it make sense to take a calf from its mother, to take a cow's milk from her baby, to take eggs from a chicken, to take chicks from their mother, to take the wool from the sheep, to take the tail from the fox? How does it make sense for anyone to poison the water, the air, the soil, and mutate the fruits, the vegetables, the nuts, the seeds, the grains or the grasses? How does it make sense to exploit other living beings to satisfy the palate or for financial gain? Especially when there are so many plant-based alternatives in almost every food store from veggie cold cuts to veggie burgers.

We are all part of one giant ecosystem. We all want our children to receive their birthrights: clean air, clean water, clean soil and clean food with love and compassion and to be able to live happy and healthy lives. We want them to continue giving these birthrights to their children and grandchildren for generations to come. Why is this concept so difficult for some to grasp and to practice? Isn't it our duty to guard, protect and nurture this beautiful creation? After all it is the only home we have!

11
Magical Godly Filters

With the way the world is today no matter how much we try to avoid being affected by environmental toxicity, still there will be different types of toxins that will penetrate our environment, our homes and our body. There are 6 major detoxification systems in our body:

THE SKIN
The largest organ and is made up of various layers. It is the protective covering of the body and protects against germs and water loss, insulates the body and helps maintain body temperature, removes toxins by sweating, takes the burden of toxins when the other systems are overloaded, gives us sensation with the help of the nerve endings it contains, absorbs a large portion of whatever it comes in contact with and is a major player in vitamin D synthesis. Some hints that the skin may needs some TLC are: acne, eczema, dry or

oily skin and blocked pores. Ideas which might be helpful in cleansing the skin include: Nourish the body with high fiber planted-based foods, fresh fruits and vegetables and healthy fats such as fresh avocados, fresh almonds, fresh ground flax seeds or cold pressed flax oil, drink plenty of pure water, use saunas, colon hydrotherapy and or enemas, chemical-free skin products and soaps and a loofah to remove old skin cells.

Juices that might be beneficial for the skin: carrot, sweet potato, turnip, onion, cucumber, wheat grass juice, apple, watermelon and grapefruit.

THE LIVER

The largest internal organ and gland of the body, is located on the right side of the body, under the diaphragm, secrets bile to break down cholesterol and toxins and metabolizes protein and carbohydrates. Some hints that the liver may need some TLC are: irritability, depression, digestive problems, high cholesterol, constipation, allergies, hypoglycemia and psoriasis. Ideas which might be helpful for cleansing the liver include: For about a week, drink first thing in the morning (at least 2 hours before eating), a mixture of: a pinch of black pepper, 1 crushed clove of garlic, 1 teaspoon of ground ginger root, 2 tablespoons of first cold pressed extra virgin olive oil and juice from at least one grapefruit and one lemon (freshly squeezed). Drink plenty of water after to wash the toxins out. Another great way to keep our liver cleansed are daily green salads made with leafy green vegetables. The greener and more bitter, usually the more cleansing. Another huge one is the green juice or the green smoothie. Juices that might be beneficial for the liver: beet, carrot, celery, lettuce, parsley, spinach, sprouts, lemon, apple, papaya, grapefruit and pineapple.

THE LARGE INTESTINE

Is found in the abdominal cavity, is made up of the cecum, colon, rectum and anal canal, absorbs water and excretes solid waste material and removes fat soluble toxins from the bile. Waste moves from the small intestine, to the cecum, the colon (about five feet long), the rectum and is released through the anus. Some hints that the large intestine may needs some TLC are: abdominal discomfort, constipation or diarrhea, irritability, headache and fatigue. Ideas which might helpful for cleansing the large intestine include: A plant-based high fiber diet, drinking plenty of clean water, making fresh fruit and vegetable smoothies – the more fiber the better, exercising, abdominal massage, enemas and colon hydrotherapy. Juices that might be beneficial for the large intestine: spinach and sweet potato.

THE LUNGS

Are found in the chest behind the rib cage on both sides of the heart, are about 11 inches long each, bring about 9500 liters of air into the body each day, oxygenate the body and remove carbon dioxide.

Some hints that the lungs may need some TLC are: hard to take deep breaths, repetitive annoying cough, feeling that mucus has a hard time coming out of the lungs, feeling congested and feeling fatigue. Ideas which might be helpful for cleansing the lungs include: clean, rich air flow to wash our lungs, deep breaths while trying to hold the air in as much as possible and trying to increase our lung capacity and elasticity, increased oxygen flow intake and carbon dioxide outtake, exercise in a clean air environment, deep breathing exercises simply by sitting straight and quietly focusing on deep breathing can be a great start, avoiding foods which may form mucus such as dairy, gluten containing foods, refined foods and sugars, consuming foods which eliminate mucus such as fresh garlic cloves and onion, avoiding toxin inhalation such as industrial air, smoking, etc., and drinking freshly squeezed hot lemonade first thing in the morning. Juices that might be beneficial for the lungs: carrot, sweet potato, kiwi and citrus.

LYMPH

Is found in the lymphatic system, made of lymphatic vessels and nodes found throughout the body and is similar to the circulatory system. Tonsils, adenoids, the spleen and appendix are part of this system. It is a colorless, clear fluid, purifies and washes the cells and carries away cellular waste through the lymphatic node filtration system. Some hints that the lymphatic system may needs some TLC are: tender, hard or swollen nodes, a tendency for infections and cellulite. Ideas for lymphatic cleansing include: exercise, trampoline jumping, using a loofah to stimulate lymphatic flow, which has a detoxifying effect, massage, taking a shower and alternating from hot to cold several times back and forth which can increase and or greatly unblock lymphatic flow and eliminating refined foods and sugars, dairy, meat and fatty food. Juices that might be beneficial for the lymphatic system: spinach.

THE KIDNEYS

Are bean-shaped organs, about 5 inches long, are located on either side of the vertebral column around the middle of the lower back, remove water soluble toxins, separate urea, mineral salts, toxins, and other waste products from the blood, conserve water, salts, and electrolytes, filter about 1800 liters of blood a day and purify the entire blood system about 10 times an hour. Some hints that the kidneys need some TLC are: dark urine, puffiness under the eyes, water retention and kidney stones. Ideas for cleansing the kidneys include: drinking enough pure water and trying to stay away from salt, alcohol and caffeine. Natural kidney cleansers include parsley, fresh asparagus, cucumber, beet, cranberries, grapes and watermelon. Watermelon is best eaten on an empty stomach and not mixed with other food to avoid gas, bloating and other digestive difficulties. Juices that might be beneficial for the kidneys: parsley, zucchini, sprouts, melon, watermelon, apple, grapefruit, apricot, plum, cherry, papaya.

Remember all the systems work hand-in-hand. That's why it is important to take the time and to care for the body as a whole. This will help all systems to work in balance and in harmony.

12

Juice Feasting

Juice feasting can be a great way to keep our filtration systems in top working condition. Our bodies are exposed to toxins all the time from the food we eat, the water we drink and the air we breathe. These toxins slowly accumulate in our system and it is important to remove them in some way. Our bodies have in-built detoxification systems, as we mentioned before, but because of our high exposure to toxins, these systems can easily become overburdened resulting in effects such as fatigue and general ill health. If these toxins are not removed the result may be chronic illness. The best way to help the body to remove excess toxins is through fasting. There are different types of fasts for different reasons. Although there are some opinions that are for water fasting, there are many who claim that water fasting releases toxins too quickly and results in a great lack of vitamins and minerals. These fasts might also cause damage to body tissues and great exhaustion. Juice fasting can be just as effective, while still providing the body with necessary vitamins, minerals and enzymes which will promote healing. (It is important to consult with a health care practitioner before attempting any fast). Remember by choosing the inexpensive fruits and vegetables, together with the fact that we don't buy other groceries during this time and we drink a lot of water, juice fasting doesn't have to be an expensive event.

So, how many days should we fast? This question has many answers. Although every day of fasting is a great healing asset, some people fast for three, five, ten, twenty one, ninety two and even a hundred days. Each set accomplishes different things. For example, a three day fast is a great detoxifier and blood cleanser and five days is an immune system strengthener. From that point and on more healing can take place having the potential to keep the body away from future illnesses.

Some say that in order to have lasting and noticeable healing results, a person should juice fast for at least 21 days. I personally experienced the benefits of juice fasting and saw the difference in effectiveness and cleansing as I progressed through the fast – from 3 days to 5 days, 10 days and finally 21 days. It is advisable to continue your daily routine, but to avoid strenuous activities as much as possible and to try to go to bed early and have at least eight hours of sleep. What happens usually while fasting is that toxins are excreted and the great amount of energy that we use for digestion is redirected to other parts of the body. These two factors help to accelerate the process of getting the body to an optimal natural state where it can rest and heal itself.

Fresh juice means using a juicer. There are no additives such as salt, sugar artificial flavors or colors. A blender is different from a juicer. While a blender blends and keeps all the ingredients, like in a smoothie, a juicer extracts the juice from the food, leaving the pulp behind. One of the advantages of juices is that they contain the purest water we can get, since the plant by itself improves and filters the water. Fresh juices have minerals, vitamins and enzymes, which are essential for healing and helping to prevent illness.

Green juice has a high amount of chlorophyll which has great healing properties. Have six to eight cups of juice a day, other than drinking water and herbal teas. During the day drink at least two liters of water. Even though you can drink it straight, many opinions say it's better to mix the juice with a third of the amount of clean, pure water. It's extremely important to keep our body slightly alkaline and not to have acidic juices like tomato, citrus juice, etc. One way to have some variation and make it easier and help with the illusion of eating is to serve the juice like a soup and eat it from a bowl. Believe it or not, it really works and you'll be surprised to discover that it's the most delicious soup you've ever eaten. Your favorite juice will usually be your favorite soup. Mine is carrot. Remember you can spice up your "juice-soup" using fresh spices such as fresh garlic or ginger or finely-ground black pepper. Potential health benefits of some popular vegetable juices: Beet juice – constipation, liver function, nerves. Cabbage juice: anti-carcinogenic, hyperthyroid, constipation and high blood pressure. Someone with hypothyroid disorder should avoid cabbage and other cruciferous vegetables. Carrot juice: liver and skin cleanser, immune and respiratory system. Celery juice: constipation, arthritis, liver function. Cucumber juice: great for high blood pressure, acne, losing weight, good for the nails, hair and skin. Lettuce juice: hair, liver function, sleeping disorders, weight loss. Parsley juice: blood purifier, diuretic, cleans the kidneys and liver. Spinach juice: bile, liver and lymphatic cleanser. Juiced sprouts: great amount of enzymes and minerals, especially alfalfa, chronic disease, fatigue, liver and kidney cleanser. Sweet potato juice: arthritis, skin, breathing and intestines. Zucchini juice: kidney cleanser. While various fruit juices can be extremely beneficial for different body systems, during a fast it is preferable to have mainly vegetable juices, since fruit juices tend to be high in sugar. It is important to dilute the juices with water or to drink water straight after drinking undiluted juices, in order to ease the work load on the kidneys. During the fast you can help to remove toxins even more effectively and accelerate the excretion of toxins by doing water enemas. Using a loofah, which is something we should try to do every day, is great advice, even more so during fasting. Also alternating hot and cold when showering is a great way to stimulate and strengthen the lymphatic system, which plays an essential part in removing waste from the cells. You may experience the effects of detoxification which can include dizziness, nausea, anxiety, dark urine or headaches. Some ideas to break the fast include having prunes that have been soaking overnight. It is still important to continue with drinking water and juices during this transition period. This can be done for a couple of days - it depends on the length of your juice feast. Then slowly introduce fruits with high water content like watermelon, etc. Next try small, frequent live fruit and vegetable meals. The easier to digest the better i.e. cut into small pieces or blended. Having cooked food right away might decrease the effects of the fast.

When you go back to eating solid food, it is best to try to avoid the following food combinations: Starch with protein or fruits. Protein with fat. Very sweet fruits with sour fruits. Fruits with vegetables. While going through the fasting process it is helpful to remember that fasting is not what actually heals; it helps the body get to the point of doing what it knows best by giving it the best conditions we can to heal itself.

13
Hydrotherapy

Although some people make funny faces when it's discussed, I think it is an important topic to mention. Everyone I know who has tried claims that it is hard to imagine life without it and wonders how come they hadn't heard about it before. It makes complete sense to clean the house's gutter or drainpipe once a year, but when it comes to our body, many people don't know where to begin, or it seems strange, weird or funny to some. When it comes to neglecting the drainpipe, if worst comes to worst, we buy a new one. When the drainpipe of the body, the colon, gets neglected and toxins and old waste accumulate, or if toxins accumulate in the liver and circulate throughout our body with the help of the circulatory system, that's a whole different story. A clean and healthy colon and liver are essential for the health of all the organs and tissues in the body. There are two types of enemas: retention and cleansing. Retention enemas are held in the body for about 15 minutes. They are used primarily to rid the liver of toxins, for example coffee or wheatgrass enemas. Cleansing enemas are retained for only a few minutes and are used to cleanse and flush the colon. An enema bag can be bought in the pharmacy for a few dollars. The 66 fluid ounce (or 2 liter) bags are a good choice. Use only chemical-free, pure water. As far as lubrication, any clean oil such as olive or coconut oil can be a good choice. Like anything else in the beginning it might feel a little uncomfortable, until you get used to using the enema. Make sure to wash and sterilize the tip and bag for next time.

To prepare your body, it's a good idea first to do an enema on an empty stomach and second to try to have only fresh juices and fluids the day before. This way it will be much easier for the waste to come out even to the level that if you weigh yourself after, you might see that you dropped a few pounds. It is also a good idea to have electrolytes such as coconut water following the enema. Colon hydrotherapy is a much more intense and effective method. It requires going to a colon hydro therapist. Typically 15 gallons of water are used to flush out the colon usually going much deeper into the colon that an enema can reach. Some of the health benefits that may be experienced following colon cleansing include: increased energy, more effective digestion, improved concentration, regularity, and increased absorption of vitamins and nutrients.

14

Sunlight

"A sun of righteousness will shine for you who honor my Name, with healing in its rays and you will go out and flourish..." (Malachi 3:20). I realized there was another big factor in my life, or life in general, that I hadn't paid enough attention to. That's right, the sun. It's pretty hard to imagine life without sunlight, but on the other hand it seems that our society today is kind of hiding from it by using artificial light, being mostly indoors, or by constantly protecting ourselves from it in any possible way. It looks like most people are afraid of having too much sun, but not of having too little. While most of us are aware of conditions that might be associated with excessive levels of sun exposure, not too many are aware of conditions that might be associated with vitamin D deficiency i.e. lower ability for calcium absorption, osteoporosis, heart disease, cervical, prostate and breast cancer, diabetes, obesity, depression and schizophrenia. We all know that all we usually need in order to get vitamin D is direct sunlight. The question is, how long should we be in the sun and what about sunscreen? Well I couldn't get a straight answer. It looks like we need to take into consideration where we live, the strength of the sun, which changes with the distance our planet is from the sun throughout the year and skin pigment. People with dark skin usually need more time in the sun than people with fair skin to absorb similar amounts of vitamin D. As far as with or without or what kind of sunscreen, there are opinions that claim that it doesn't matter what kind or strength you are using, you will hardly be able to absorb any vitamin D. Other than that what about the possible risk of absorbing all the chemicals into your skin especially when the pores are wide open with the heat of the sun? Some say that 10 minutes a day with direct sun and no lotion might be a good start. As far as winter or places with very little sunlight, vitamin D3 supplementation might be the way to go. A good idea is to take a blood test to check your vitamin D3 level before and if needed after taking the supplement.

15
Fitness

"By the sweat of your brow shall you eat bread…" (Genesis 3:19).

Exercising such as stretching, walking, running, playing ball and swimming are activities that cause us joy.

Believe it or not, even going on the swing in the playground and climbing on the jungle gym can be a fun and great workout. What I found is that playing in the playground, connects us to the child within us and in a magical way can make us feel younger. The Rambam in his medical books explains that we need to really search for a type of exercise which wakes up the soul more than one that wakes up the body. An easier and more pleasant way to do this is by playing ball. Playing with a small ball is better than other exercise and has less risk of injury than other types of sport.

By strengthening the spirit for example by laughing, the body is strengthened and its natural warmth increases. He explains that exercise is any movement that causes a person to change his breathing pattern to a faster and stronger one than being at rest. However excessive and intense exercise like weightlifting can cause the body to be tight and dry and the mind to become stagnant. Also when a person feels that he worked hard and is tired and feels hot, that is a good time to stop working out. It looks like there are three major areas in exercise stretching, cardio and weights. To maximize their benefits they should all be done with joy.

16

Intimacy

Just like excessive and intense exercise can dry and damage the body, excessive intimate relations can also cause damage since it squeezes out the natural humidity of the body. We have mentioned how to obtain energy and life force through sleep, sun and foods such as fruits, vegetables, nuts and seeds. Roots such as garlic, ginger, carrots, beet, etc. contain the essence of the plant and it's vitalizing force. The same applies to nuts and seeds, which are concentrated energy sources. When it comes to humans, the vitalizing force is found in the "seed", the sperm. Just like we need to take in life force in order to have life force, we need to preserve life force in order to keep it. So how can we go about preserving this life force? There is an interesting answer in the following text, which was written about

800 years ago. "Semen is the strength of the body, its life force, and the light of the eyes; the greater the emission of sperm, the more damages to the body, to its strength and the greater the loss to one's longevity…Therefore, a person must take care in this matter if he wishes to live in good health. He should not engage in intercourse except when the body is healthy and particularly strong, when he has many involuntary erections…Such a person needs to engage in intercourse and it is medically advisable. He should not engage in intercourse on a full or empty stomach, but after the food has been digested. He should examine himself to see if he needs to move his bowels or urinate before and after intercourse. He should not engage in intercourse while standing or sitting, nor in the bathhouse…Whoever is constantly involved in sexual relations, old age comes upon him before its time, his strength is depleted, his eyes become dim, a bad odor comes from his mouth and his armpits, the hair of his head, his eyebrows, and eyelashes fall out, the hair of his beard, armpits, and legs grows in abundance, his teeth fall out and he suffers many pains beyond these. The wise of the doctors have said: One of a thousand dies from other illnesses and a thousand from excessive intercourse" (Rambam Deot 4:19).

17

Centenarians & Longevity

The Torah tells us that for twenty generations from creation to Abraham, people lived for hundreds of years with Methuselah being the oldest recorded person at 969 years old, "And all the days of Methuselah were nine hundred and sixty nine years, and he died" (Genesis 5:27). Even though from the time of Abraham life expectancy actually decreased dramatically centenarians were still very common both among men and women. "Sarah's lifetime was one hundred years, twenty years and seven years; the years of Sarah's life" (Genesis 23:1). "Now these are the days of the years of Abraham's life which he lived: a hundred years, seventy years, and five years" (Genesis 25:1). "Isaac's days were one hundred and eighty years" (Genesis 35:28). "…and the days of Jacob – the years of his life - were one hundred and forty-seven years" (Genesis 47:28). "Joseph died at the end of one hundred and ten years…" (Genesis 50:26). "Aaron was one hundred and twenty-three years old at his death on Mount Hor" (Numbers 33:39). "Moses was one hundred and twenty years old when he died; his eye had not dimmed, and his vigor had not diminished" (Deuteronomy 34:7). The list goes on.

In those days people lived in tribes meaning they were surrounded by family and relatives. Their family and relatives were their identity. The tribe of Judah meant that they were all children of Judah. The tribe of Levi meant that they were all children of Levi and so on. Living this way, people were not afraid to be alone. People were not afraid to get older and age alone. They were not afraid to be put in a nursing home to be alone and forgotten. They knew that their family would be around them until the last moment. More than that being old meant being wise and was considered to be noble and respected. It is mentioned in the Torah to stand up in front of the elderly, "In the presence of an old person you shall rise…" (Leviticus 19:32) and is rooted in one of the Ten Commandments, "Honor your father and your mother, so that your days will be lengthened upon the land that Hashem, your God, gives you" (Exodus 20:12).

People were much more social. They were not entertained by digital screens but by their family and friends. They danced, sang and worked together. The family's love and affection surrounded the person. While the early generations did not eat any animal products at all, in later generations when meat was eaten, it was eaten very rarely. There were many rules associated with eating meat such as where, how much and for how long it could be eaten. People would go for days in the desert with water and dried fruits. Staple foods were grains such as wheat, barley, millet and spelt. Legumes like lentils were also very popular as well as dried fruits, nuts and seeds. "So Abraham hastened to the tent to Sarah and said, "Hurry! Three se'ahs of meal, fine flour! Knead and make cakes!" (Genesis 18:6). "Israel their father said to them, "…Take of the land's glory in your baggage and bring it down to the man as a tribute –a bit of balsam, a bit of honey, wax, lotus, pistachios, and almonds" (Genesis 43:11). "And you, take yourself wheat and barley, and beans and lentils, and millet and spelt…" (Ezekiel 4:9). Of course the food was locally grown, organic, non GMO, etc. In those days people were active. They walked everywhere and did everything with their hands. Being sedentary was rare.

There was respect for nature and natural resources. People lived and understood the importance of a tree for its shade, for its fruit. "When you besiege a city for many days to wage war against it to capture it, you shall not destroy its trees by wielding an ax against them, for you may eat from them, but you shall not cut them down…" (Deuteronomy 20:19). There was no need for environmental conservation. It was an instinct. People lived with nature and with animals. It was a way of life. There was no need for pets as companions. There were no factories or cars or other major sources of air pollution.

People got enough sunshine. They were outdoors getting their vitamin D on a regular basis without being afraid of ozone depletion. The soil was fertile and not depleted. Food was nutrient dense and was not lacking. All fertilizers were natural and organic. It looks like permaculture was a lifestyle. People lived in tents and were nomadic. They didn't worry about a mortgage or paying bills. Each person had a place to live and food to eat. If they had to leave for some reason, they simply packed their belongings and left. Later, after entering the Land, each person was allocated a lot of land according to the size of their family. Obviously there were other worries, but it seems like the foundation was healthier and more solid.

It's interesting that there are still places and cultures in the world today such as Okinawa in Japan, Vilcabamba in Ecuador, the Hunza people in Pakistan and Abkhasia people of Caucasus in southern Russia, where people are still living according to many of the above values. Not surprisingly these people have the highest number of healthy, active and clear-minded centenarians in the world and terminal, western diseases are rare or unknown. It seems that people have always been fascinated with longevity and the search for the "fountain of youth". How many potions and formulas, how much research and how many books have been written about longevity and living a healthy lifestyle? While people have been searching for the right formula of how to live and eat, the Torah has been teaching us this wisdom for thousands of years. So what's next?

So of course "in His hand is the soul of every living thing and the spirit of all mankind" (Job 12:10), but it is in our hands to learn more about creation and its laws and how to connect in a better, healthier, spiritual and physical way to the Source and it's rhythm – it's endless. On the physical level we can start by growing our own organic fruits and vegetables, starting with indoor gardening and then slowly moving towards growing outdoors, with the goal of becoming as self-sustainable as possible. We can continue with solar energy, by putting solar panels to use for hot water, heating and electricity, which can help reduce pollution, bring the creation closer to the way it was meant to be and hopefully help our pocket as well. There is always more to be done. The "permaculture" ecosystem can be a great help, since the whole approach is about respecting and living in harmony with creation.

18

Crystals

Rabbi Shimon the son of Yochai says that a precious stone hung from Abraham our forefather's neck and every sick person that saw it was instantly healed and when Abraham our forefather passed away, Hashem hung the stone in the sun (Baba Batra 16:2). The Talmud explains that in his life, this precious stone was close to him. Now it hangs in the sky of all, it is within the sun itself "sun, kindness and healing"(Malachi 3:20). "You shall make a "choshen" (breastplate) of judgment, the work of a master weaver. You shall make it like the work of the ephod; of gold, blue, purple, and scarlet wool, and twisted fine linen shall you make it. It shall be square doubled; its length a half cubit and its width a half cubit. And you shall fill into it stone fillings, four rows of stones. One row: Odem, Pitdah, and Bareketh; thus shall the one row be. The second row: Nofech, Sappir, and Yahalom. The third row: Leshem, Shevo, and Achlamah. And the fourth row: Tarshish, Shoham, and Yashpheh; they shall be set in gold in their fillings. And the stones shall be according to the names of the sons of Israel twelve, corresponding to their names; the engravings of a seal, every one according to his name shall they be, for the twelve tribes" (Exodus 28:15-21).

Rabbi Bechaiyeh (Rabbi and kabbalist, Spain, 1255-1340) says that there are 12 major stones that are the root of all the precious stones. All the other precious stones are derived from them. The first stone "Odem" for the tribe of Reuven is the ruby - a red stone, and is found in known places in the sea. A pregnant woman who carries it shouldn't have a miscarriage. It is also good for a woman who has difficulty giving birth and if the rock is ground and mixed with food or drink it is very helpful for pregnancy, just like the jasmine flowers that Reuven found (Genesis 14-17). The second stone "Pitdah" for the tribe of Shimon is a green and shiny rock. It cools the body. It's found in the countries of "Cush", (Ethiopia according to some people). "The pitdah of Cush cannot be approximated; the purest gold cannot be compared to it" (Job 28:19). The third stone "Bareketh" for the tribe of Levi sparkles like lightening and shines like a candle. It was given to the tribe of Levi because they "shone" in Torah and also when Moses, from the tribe of Levi, was born the whole house was filled with light. It also says that when Moses came down from the mountain the skin of his face shone with light. It says in Ecclesiastes: "…a man's wisdom illuminates his face…" (Ecclesiastes 8:1). This stone helps people to be wiser and less naïve. By grinding it and mixing it with food and drink, it will benefit a person by opening the heart and becoming wiser. The fourth stone "Nofech" for the tribe of Yehudah is a green stone. We have seen the multiple victories of the tribe of Judah and the most famous one is the victory of King David. Whoever wears this stone, his enemies turn away. "Your hand is in the neck of your enemies" (Genesis 49:8).

The fifth stone "Sappir" for the tribe of Yissachar is blue. It's the color of humility and it's good for the eyes. That's why some people pass it over the eyes, just like the Torah illuminates the eyes. It was given to the tribe of Yissachar because they were known for their knowledge of Torah and the actual tablets were made from "snappirinon". It's also good for pain and inflammation in the body, just like the Torah heals the entire body. "And Moses and Aaron, Nadab and Abihu, and seventy of the elders of Israel ascended, and they perceived the God of Israel, and beneath His feet was like the forming of a sapphire ("Sappir") brick and like the appearance of the heavens for clarity" (Exodus 24:9-10). The sixth stone "Yahalom" for the tribe of Zevulun is white, just like silver is white. It's the sign for the wealth of the tribe of Zevulun, which was known for commerce. This stone is good for success in business and is helpful in falling asleep. The seventh stone "Leshem" for the tribe of Dan is from the passage in the book of Joshua "...and changed the name of "Leshem" to Dan..." (Joshua 19:47). The eighth stone "Shevo" for the tribe of Naftali is called "turquoisa". People who ride horses carry it. It connects the person to a vehicle and brings success in riding a vehicle. The ninth stone "Achlamah" for the tribe of Gad is reddish. It strengthens the heart from fear and is from the Hebrew word "chozek" (strength). The tenth stone "Tarshish" for the tribe of Asher is the color of oil or the color of the sea. It's good for digestion.

The eleventh stone "Shoham" for the tribe of Yosef to find favor with others. Whoever carries it in the house of leadership, his words will be heard. The twelve stone "Yashpheh" for the tribe of Binyamin is made up of many shades, red, black and green. It's good to stop bleeding. These twelve precious stones which were in the Breastplate were according to the order of their birth, tribe by tribe. Rabbi Bechayeh (Spain, 1255-1340) read in a book that these stones need purification and it's known that if whoever carries them is impure, the stones' properties become weaker or will diminish completely. And by the person purifying himself, the properties of the stones will come back. This is because the spiritual levels and the supreme power that the rock nourishes from cleaves to purity and distances itself from impurity...(Rabbeinu Bechayeh commentary on the Torah, Exodus 28:15. See the source for the full, detailed and fascinating explanation). Another opinion as to the stones found in the Breastplate is as follows: The first row in the Breastplate: "Odem" a ruby for the tribe of Reuven, "Pitdah" an emerald for Shimon, "Bareketh" a topaz for Levi. The second row: "Nofech" a carbuncle for Judah, "Sappir" a sapphire for Yissachar, "Yahalom" a quartz crystal for Zevulun. The third row: "Leshem" a jacinth for Dan, "Shevo" an agate for Naftali, "Achlamah" an amethyst for Gad. The fourth and last row: "Tarshish" a chrysolite for Asher, "Shoham" an onyx for Yosef, "Yashpheh" an opal for Binyamin (Carta's Illustrated Encyclopedia of the Holy Temple in Jerusalem).

There is a famous commentary on the story when Joshua lost the war at the "Ai" (Joshua 7:1-19). Hashem told Joshua that one of the reasons they lost was because someone had taken from the consecrated property, which they had been commanded not to take. Joshua succeeded to locate the person. The commentary explains that this was done using the crystals in the "choshen" (breastplate of the "kohen gadol" (high priest) on which there was a crystal representing each of the tribes. When the responsible tribe passed in front of the "choshen", the crystal that represented the responsible tribe dimmed. When the people of the tribe walked in front of it, the same stone dimmed as the responsible person passed by.

All crystals other than amber, coral and pearl are a combination of minerals that were created with high temperatures and pressure of the earth utilizing the minerals that were around. The crystallization process is very slow forming one cell after another in a precise and defined way. During this process the crystal accumulates great energy which is the source of its properties and consciousness. We know that the quartz can transmit electric impulses. The energy emitted from a crystal has been documented many times as a white aura coming out from the middle of it. This energy is claimed to have healing properties.

19
Color Therapy

There are many examples of the importance of color descriptions and uses in the Torah: "Hashem spoke to Moses saying: "Speak to the children of Israel, and have them take for Me an offering; from every person whose heart inspires him to generosity, you shall take My offering. And this is the offering that you shall take from them: gold, silver, and copper; blue, purple, and crimson wool…" (Exodus 25:1-4). "And the Mishkan (Tabernacle) you shall make out of ten curtains of twisted fine linen, and blue, purple, and crimson wool. A cheruvim design of the work of a master weaver you shall make them" (Exodus 26:1). "And you shall make a dividing curtain of blue, purple, and crimson wool, and twisted fine linen; the work of a master weaver he shall make it, in a cheruvim design" (Exodus 26:31).

"Mordechai left the king's presence clad in royal apparel of turquoise and white with a large gold crown and a robe of fine linen and purple. Then the city of Shushan was cheerful and glad" (Esther 8:15). I believe that everything happens for a reason. It's no coincidence that we see the world in color. Just like the precious stones on the high priest's breastplate affected our life, in the same way, every stone and its color was chosen in a very precise way for each of the twelve tribes. Just like it wasn't a coincidence that the Tabernacle was described in detail for each and every color and its location. And just like when Hashem spoke to Moses and said: "Speak to the children of Israel and you shall say to them that they shall make for themselves fringes on the corners of their garments, throughout their generations, and they shall affix a thread of sky blue on the fringe of each corner" (Numbers 15:38). It was not a coincidence that the color blue was chosen. "Our sages say that sky blue is similar to the color of the sea, the sea to the sky and the sky to Hashem's throne of Glory" (Menachot 43b).

If we look carefully around us we can probably figure out a few helpful uses of colors in our everyday life. For instance: Blue is a cold color. That's why it is relaxing and calming and may help with lowering blood pressure and reducing pain and inflammation. That's why in summer it might be a good idea to surround ourselves with blue, for example, our linen and clothes, as this could have a cooling effect. Green is similar to blue. Just like walking in a green environment is very relaxing and calming and is a mood enhancer, a similar effect might be achieved by surrounding ourselves with this color. Red on the other hand is a warm color. That's why it's stimulating and may be helpful in increasing blood flow and blood pressure. That's why in the winter time it might be a good idea to surround ourselves with red, for example, using red blankets and sweaters, as this could have a warming effect. Red could be a good color for someone who is a little frigid, lacks energy or who has anemia. Pink has a soothing effect. It can benefit anxious or aggressive people. Yellow is a good color for memory. That's why some study books are printed on yellow paper. Yellow is also the color of the sun. Just like the sun gives vitality to the planet, we might be affected in a similar way by surrounding ourselves with this color. There are many more colors and shades but it all comes down to the same thing: be in touch with creation and listen to its rhythm.

20
Music Therapy

"You should know that every shepherd has its own melody according to the grasses and the location where he is tending...because every grass has its own melody which it says...and from the melodies of the grasses it becomes a melody of a shepherd" (Likutei Moharan II 63). "If you were to merit to hear the voice of the grasses praising how each one is saying poetry to Hashem blessed be He, with no complaints or foreign thoughts and without expectation for a reward, how beautiful and graceful it is when their singing is heard and it's great to worship Hashem with awe among them" (Sichot Haran 273). "It's good for a person to get into the habit of reviving himself with a holy melody because a melody is extremely high spiritually and it has a great power to bring and continue the human heart to Hashem blessed be He"(Sichot Haran 273). I remember playing the guitar in the park one day. Suddenly my wife and I saw raccoons coming down the trees and slowly approaching us another one and another one. First they came from trees around us, and then from farther and farther away. We couldn't figure out why. At first we thought that they thought we had food, which we didn't. Then we thought maybe we were in their territory, which we weren't. Then we started to feel threatened like we were experiencing a raccoon attack so we got into the car and left. Later after telling the story to a park ranger, she started laughing asking surprisingly, "Don't you know that animals love music?" It made so much sense. After all, who doesn't like music?

It is a real thing that listening to music can help with healing. It can help the brain to release the feel good chemical dopamine, it can affect our heart rate, our breathing patterns and assist in relaxing and opening our blood vessels. Music together with a soothing voice and positive words can be even more effective. It is even possible to see pictures of how water molecules change shape with music and kind words. Here are some examples of how music was used in the biblical days:

MUSIC & CELEBRATIONS

"Now all the work that Solomon did for the House of the Hashem was completed and Solomon brought his father David's hallowed things, and the silver and the gold and all the vessels he deposited in the treasuries of the House of Hashem...And the Levites who sang-all of them, Asaph, Heman, Jeduthun, and their sons and their brethren, attired in fine linen, with cymbals and with psalteries and with harps, standing east of the altar, and with them were priests one hundred twenty sounding with trumpets. And the trumpeters and the singers were as one, to make one sound, to praise and to thank Hashem, and when they raised a sound with trumpets and with cymbals and with the musical instruments and with praise to the Hashem, "for He is good, because His kindness is eternal," and the House became full of the cloud of the House of Hashem. And the priests could not stand to serve because of the cloud, because the glory of Hashem filled the House of Hashem" (Chronicles II 5:1, 12-14).

MUSIC & HEALING DEPRESSION

"Samuel took the horn of oil, and anointed him in the midst of his brothers. And a spirit of Hashem passed over David from that day forth. Then Samuel arose and went to Ramah. And the spirit of Hashem departed from Saul, and he was tormented by a spirit of melancholy from Hashem. And Saul's servants said to him, "Behold now, a spirit of melancholy from God torments you. Let our lord tell your servants before you they should seek a man who knows how to play on the harp so that when the spirit of melancholy is upon you he will play with his hand, and it will be good for you." So Saul said to his servants, "Seek now for me someone who plays well, and bring him to me." One of the young servants spoke up and said, "Behold, I saw a son of Jesse the Bethlehemite, who knows how to play, a mighty man of valor, and a man of war, and who understands a matter, and is a handsome man, and Hashem is with him." Saul sent messengers to Jesse, and he said, "Send me David your son, who is with the sheep." And Jesse took a donkey laden with bread, and a jug of wine, and one kid and he sent them with David his son, to Saul. And David came to Saul, and stood before him, and he loved him very much, and he was his weapon bearer. And Saul sent to Jesse, saying, "Let David stand before me now, for he has found favor in my eyes." And it would be, that when the spirit of melancholy was upon Saul, that David would take the harp, and would play with his hand, and Saul would be relieved, and it would be good for him, and the spirit of melancholy would depart from him" (Samuel I 16: 13-23).

MUSIC & CONNECTING TO THE DIVINE

"And Jehoshaphat said, "Is there no prophet of Hashem here that we may inquire of Hashem through him?" And one of the king of Israel's servants answered, "Here is Elisha the son of Shaphat, who poured water on Elijah's hands." And Jehoshaphat said, "The word of Hashem is with him." And the king of Israel and Jehoshaphat and the king of Edom went down to him. And Elisha said to the king of Israel, "What do we have to do with one another? Go to your father's prophets and to your mother's prophets! "And the king of Israel said to him, "Don't say that, for Hashem has summoned these three kings to deliver them into the hands of Moab." And Elisha said, "As Hashem Master of Legions, before Whom I have stood, lives, for were it not that I respect Jehoshaphat king of Judah, I would neither look at you nor would I see you. And now bring me a musician." And it was that when the musician played, the hand of Hashem came upon him" (Kings II 3:11-15).

MUSICAL INSTRUMENTS IN SCRIPTURE

LUTE (KINOR) & WIND OR STRING INSTRUMENT (UGAV) (ORGAN IN MODERN HEBREW)
"And his brother's name was Jubal; he was the father of all who grasp a lute and ugav" (Genesis 4:21).

DRUM (TOF) & LUTE (KINOR)
"Why have you fled secretly, and concealed from me, and not told me? I would have sent you away with joy

and with songs, with drum and lute" (Genesis 31:27).

TIMBREL (TOF)

"Miriam, the prophetess, Aaron's sister, took a timbrel in her hand, and all the women came out after her with timbrels and with dances" (Exodus 15:20).

SHOFAR

"The sound of the shofar grew increasingly stronger; Moses would speak and God would answer him with a voice" (Exodus 19:19).

"You shall proclaim with the shofar blasts, in the seventh month, on the tenth of the month; on the Day of Atonement, you shall sound the shofar throughout your land" (Leviticus 25:9).

TRUMPETS (HATZOTZROT)

"Make yourself two silver trumpets; you shall make them from a beaten form; they shall be used by you to summon the congregation and to announce the departure of the camps" (Numbers 10:2).

TRIANGLES (SHALISHIM)

"...the women came out of all the cities of Israel, to sing, and with musical instruments in their hands, toward King Saul, with drums, with joy, and with triangles" (Samuel I 18:6).

HARPS (NEVALIM), SISTRA (MENAANEIM) & TZELTZELIM (SMALL CYMBALS)

"And David and all the house of Israel were rejoicing with all kinds of cypress-woods, with lutes, and with harps, and with drums, and with sistra, and with small cymbals" (Samuel II 6:5).

FLUTE (HALIL)

"And there are lute and harp, drum and flute…"(Isaiah 5:12).

SHEMINIT (INSTRUMENT WITH 8 STRINGS)

"To the conductor with melodies on the sheminit, a song of David" (Psalms 6:1).

WHISTLING HORN (MASHROKITA) CLAVICHORD (KATROS) & BAGPIPES (SUMPONIA)

"At the time that you hear the sound of the whistling horn, the clavichord, the harp, the psaltery, the bagpipes, and all kinds of music…" (Daniel 3:5).

COPPER CYMBALS (METZILTAYIM NEHOSHET)

"And the singers: Heman, Asaph, and Ethan, with copper cymbals to resound" (Chronicles I 15:19).

CYMBALS (METZILTAYIM)

"And the Levites who sang-all of them, Asaph, Heman, Jeduthun, and their sons and their brethren, attired in fine linen, with cymbals and with harps and with lutes, standing east of the altar, and with them were priests-one hundred twenty sounding with trumpets" (Chronicles II 5:12).

SINGING (ZIMRA)

"Raise song and give forth a drum, a pleasant lute with a harp" (Psalms 81:3).

Voice and singing are infinite instruments: they have so many different sounds, tunes, melodies, voices, accents, phrases, words, letters, vowels etc. We can see a great example in the book of Psalms and Song of Songs with so many poets, musicians and choices of words. Some words are repeated more often than others usually at the beginning of the psalm like: halleluyah, song, give thanks, ascents, for the conductor, a prayer, a psalm, sing joyfully etc.

Since the Bible did not come with an audio CD these repeating words are like hint instruments meaning if we know it's a give thanks song it will have a different melody from a prayer song, etc. That's why if we contemplate on these words and listen carefully, we might be able to hear the original ancient melodies that were playing thousands of years ago.

21

The Divine & Interior Design

There are many sayings from different sources which claim spiritual and mystical benefits of specific locations and directions such as: It is written that east is where light comes out to the world, west is the mouth, north is hearing and south is smell (Zohar Tikun 70). Whoever wants to get richer should go north and whoever wants to gain wisdom should go south. There is also an idea not to place the bed with the feet facing towards the door since that was the customary way to place deceased people. The place where we find actual Divine instruction about where to place each item is in the story of the Tabernacle in the book of Exodus. After five long, creative and detailed chapters the Torah puts emphasis on how everything was built and placed, as Hashem commanded, resulting in the cloud covering the Tent of Meeting, and the glory of Hashem filling up the Tabernacle: "It was in the first month of the second year on the first of the month that the Tabernacle was set up. Moses set up the Tabernacle; he put down its sockets and emplaced its planks and inserted its bars, and set up its pillars. He spread the Tent over the Tabernacle and put the Cover of the Tent on it from above, as Hashem had commanded Moses.

He took and placed the Testimony into the Ark and inserted the staves on the Ark, and he placed the Cover on the Ark from above. He brought the Ark into the Tabernacle and emplaced the Partition sheltering the Ark of Testimony, as Hashem had commanded Moses. He put the Table in the Tent of Meeting on the north side of the Tabernacle, outside the Partition. He prepared on it the setting of bread before Hashem, as Hashem had commanded Moses. He placed the Menorah in the Tent of Meeting, opposite the Table, on the south side of the Tabernacle. He kindled the lamps before Hashem, as Hashem had commanded Moses. He placed the Gold Altar in the Tent of Meeting, in front of the Partition. Upon it he caused incense spices to go up in smoke, as Hashem had commanded Moses. He emplaced the Curtain of the entrance of the Tabernacle. He placed the Elevation-offering Altar at the entrance of the Tent of Meeting, and brought up upon it the elevation-offering and the meal-offering, as Hashem had commanded Moses. He emplaced the Laver (a big basin for water) between the Tent of Meeting and the Altar, and there he put water for washing. Moses, Aaron, and his sons washed their hands and feet from it. When they came to the Tent of Meeting and when they approached the Altar they would wash, as Hashem had commanded Moses. He set up the Courtyard all around the Tabernacle and the Altar, and he emplaced the curtain of the gate of the Courtyard. So Moses completed the work. The cloud covered the Tent of Meeting, and the glory of Hashem filled the Tabernacle" (Exodus 40:17-35).

There is an interesting story in the Zohar about a mystical handicapped person, who by saying the special 52-letter name of Hashem found himself together with two wise ones at the entrance to a special cave. Then the Zohar describes the objects inside and their location in detail. Obviously there are many deep mystical meanings behind it, but on a simple level the description is as follows: A table to the left with all the delicacies of the world on it. A lamp with seven candles to the south. A silver, gold and precious stone bed to the west between north and south and a chair to the east (Tikunea haZohar, Tikun 69). The story continues with a description of more chambers with other interesting objects.

22
Purity & Jewish Monks (Nazirites)

The Torah explains that "Only a spring or a cistern (an underground reservoir for rainwater), a gathering of water, shall remain pure…"(Leviticus 11:36).

Although the disqualification of drawn water is a rabbinic decree, our Sages explained it based on an association found in a Biblical verse. Leviticus states: "Only a spring, a cistern, or a gathering of water shall be pure." Based on a comparison of the terms used in the verse, they explained: The water of "a spring" is not dependent on man's activity at all. The water of "a cistern" is entirely dependent on man's activity, for it contains drawn water entirely. Our Sages said: The "gathering of water" should not be entirely made up of drawn water like a cistern, nor need it come entirely from the

Hand of Heaven. Instead, if it came into being partially through human effort, it is acceptable.) (Rambam Mikvaot 4:1, 2). The Sages explained the gathering of water should contain enough water for the entire body of a human being to immerse in it at one time. They measured this figure as a cubit by a cubit by a height of three cubits. This measure contains 40 se'ah of water (648-750 liters – Chazon Ish; 554.283 - 921.6 liters – Rabbi Avraham Chaim). According to Rabbinic Law, water that is drawn is invalid for immersion. Moreover, if there was a body of water less than 40 se'ah that was not drawn and three lugim (biblical measure) of drawn water fell into it, the entire body of water is invalidated. All impure entities - whether humans or vessels, regain purity only through immersion in water that is collected in a pool in the ground (Rambam Mikvaot 1:1).

There are six categories of "mikveot" (purification baths) one superior to another: The first is water in a pit, water storage tanks, storage trenches, storage caverns, and the like, where water is collected on the earth...The second level is rainwater that has not ceased flowing, i.e., the rain is still descending and the mountains are still gushing with water and that water flows down and collects on the ground. It is not "drawn". However, there are not 40 se'ah...The third level is a "mikveh" that contains 40 se'ah of water that was not drawn... The fourth level is a natural spring whose water is minimal and drawn water was added to it…The fifth level is a natural spring in which drawn water was not mixed, but its water was spoiled; it was bitter or salty…The sixth and highest level is a natural spring whose water is "living water"…(Rambam Mikvaot ch. 9). In case a man cannot immerse in a ritual bath there is a custom, to continuously pour 13.5 liters (9 kabin) of water straight on their head in the shower in order to become purified. If for some reason this is also impossible, he can wash his hands forty times using a vessel with a special order and intentions (Rav Pealim, Sod Yesharim, part 4:3 by the Ben Ish Chai, Rabbi, master kabbalist and authority on Jewish law, Babylon, 1832-1909).

Another custom: "Since every man upon rising from his bed in the morning is like a newborn creation, for the worship of the Creator, Blessed be His name, so he needs to sanctify himself and wash his hands from a vessel, like the "cohen" (priest) used to sanctify by washing his hands daily out of the wash-basin before performing his temple service" (Kitzur Shulchan Aruch, Netilat Yadayim 2:1,9).

"…Torah leads to watchfulness (zehirut), watchfulness leads to quickness (zrizut), quickness leads to cleanliness (nekiut), cleanliness leads to abstention (prishut), abstention leads to purity (tahara), purity leads to piety (hasidut), piety leads to humility (anava), humility leads to fear of wrongdoing (yirat het), fear of wrongdoing leads to holiness (kedusha), holiness leads to prophecy (nevuah)..."(Avodah Zarah 20b). One example of a purer life style were the nazirites (Jewish monks) who consecrated themselves to the service of God, under very specific vows: "Hashem spoke to Moses saying: Speak to the children of Israel, and you shall say to them: A man or woman who sets himself apart by making a nazirite vow to abstain for the sake of Hashem. He shall abstain from new wine and aged wine; he shall not drink even vinegar made from new wine or aged wine, nor shall he drink anything in which grapes have been steeped, and he shall eat neither fresh grapes nor dried ones.

For the entire duration of his abstinence, he shall not eat any product of the grape vine, from seeds to skins. All the days of his vow of abstinence, no razor shall pass over his head; until the completion of the term that he abstains for the sake of Hashem, it shall be sacred, and he shall allow the growth of the hair of his head to grow wild. All the days that he abstains for Hashem, he shall not come into contact with the dead. To his father, to his mother, to his brother, or to his sister, he shall not defile himself if they die, for the crown of his God is upon his head. For the entire duration of his abstinence, he is holy to Hashem" (Numbers 6:1-8). Two well known examples of nazirites were:

Samuel: "And Hannah arose after eating and after drinking, and Eli the priest was sitting on the chair beside the doorpost of the Temple of Hashem. And she was bitter in spirit, and she prayed to Hashem, and wept. And she vowed a vow, and said: to Master of Legions, if You will look upon the affliction of Your bondswoman, and You will remember me, and You will not forget Your bondswoman and You will give Your bondswoman a man-child, and I shall give him to Hashem all the days of his life, and no razor shall come upon his head...And it was, when the time came about, after Hannah had conceived, that she bore a son, and she called his name Samuel, because she said, "I asked him of Hashem" (Samuel I 1:9-11, 20). And Samuel was serving before Hashem, being a lad girded with a linen robe. And the lad, Samuel, was growing up, and bettering himself both with Hashem and with people (Samuel I 2:18, 26). And Hashem continued to appear in Shiloh, for Hashem revealed Himself to Samuel in Shiloh with the word of Hashem" (Samuel I 3:21). Samson: "And an angel of Hashem appeared to the woman, and said to her, "Behold now, you are barren, and have not borne; and you shall conceive and bear a son. Consequently, beware now, and do not drink wine or strong drink, and do not eat any unclean thing. Because you shall conceive, and bear a son; and a razor shall not come upon his head, for a Nazirite to God shall the lad be from the womb; and he will begin to save Israel..." (Judges 13:3-5).

23

Ancient Meditation

It is explained that the early righteous ones would clear their mind from the matters of this world and connect their mind to the Almighty with love and fear. For nine hours they would put their learning aside for "hitbodedut" and contemplation, meditating that the Light of the Divine Presence was upon their heads, spreading around them, with them sitting in its center. And then they would naturally start shaking and that shaking would bring them great joy, since they could fulfill the verse in Psalms (2:11) "Serve Hashem with awe, and rejoice with trembling" (The book of Haredim end of ch. 65).

"Hitbodedut", "prishut" and "dvekut" used to be a custom of the Sages meaning while being by themselves, separating their mind from matters of this world and connecting their thoughts with the Master of all. And so it was taught by my teacher the kabbalist that this can benefit the soul seven times more than learning. According to the strength and ability of a person he should do so once a week, once in fifteen days or once a month, but not less" (The Book of Haredim, ch. 65). Another method is for a person to picture himself as a seat for holiness and imagine that on top of each organ of his body, Hashem's Name is placed in different spelling and vowel variations, according to the ten Divine attributes (details can be found in "Edot Hamizrah" prayer books).

24

Character Detox

All the undesirable characteristics are rooted in the four levels of the fundamental soul from the bad side and from the shell "klipah" that is within it. Therefore all the undesirable characteristics are divided into four types as follows: The element of fire is pride or rudeness which is drawn from it, being the lightest and the "tallest". It includes anger since as a result of pride a person becomes angry when people don't do his will, and if he were humble and knew his shortcomings then he wouldn't get angry at all. The conclusion is that pride and anger are one characteristic. Its three outcomes are: a) being critical in his heart, since without pride he wouldn't criticize in his heart, just like we explained about anger; b) looking for power and honor, to be vain towards the creations; and c) dislike towards others for being greater than him which comes from the branch of pride as well. The element of wind is the place where speech or pointless talks (general, spiritual or physical) are drawn from. Its four outcomes are: speech of flattery, lies, slander and to boast to others. The element of water is the place where lust for pleasures is drawn from since from water grows all kinds of pleasure. Its two outcomes are a) coveting to steal his friend's money and wife and whatever he has for lustful purposes; and b) jealousy that he will be jealous of his friend who has great wealth for lustful purposes.

The element of earth is the place where sadness and all its aspects are drawn from. It has one outcome which is the laziness to fulfill Torah and it's commandments "mitzvot" because of his sadness about not obtaining futile, physical possessions of this world or because of the hardships which come upon him and not being happy in his share in anything, also his eyes will never be satisfied by wealth.

It's concluded that the roots of all the undesirable characteristics are four: a) pride and anger which is included and cleaves to it "gaava" b) pointless talk "sicha beteila" c) lust for pleasures "taavot vetaanugim" d) sadness "atzvut". The four of them are drawn from the four shells "klipot" of the evil inclination that is in the fundamental soul. Their opposites are the four good characteristics which are drawn from the four foundations of good, which are in the fundamental soul, and they are: a) humility "anava", which keeps the person away from all kinds of anger which come as a result of pride "gaava", b) silence "shtika", as a mute person who wouldn't open his mouth other than for matters of Torah and commandments "mitzvot" or for what is necessary for the existence of the body and for the respect of the creations, c) disgust "mioot taavot" from all bodily lust for pleasures, being satisfied with little, d) constant happiness "simcha" with his share, because everything from Heaven is for good. Also to be quick and extremely happy serving his Creator as it says in Psalms 119: "I rejoice over your word, like one who finds abundant spoils" and like the Sages said: "Make the Torah your permanent occupation…"(Avot a:15).

"…And when he will overcome his inclination and fight it and will remove his undesirable characteristics through hard work and will fulfill Torah and commandments "mitzvot" he will be called a completely righteous person, God-fearing, a hero who conquered his inclination. And when he will practice it and get used to it for some time…then he will be enclothed with the four letters of Hashem's Name and will become a "holy chair" (dwelling place) for His chariot blessed be He. This person is named "loving Hashem from love" and is called completely righteous…" (Shaarei Kedusha part 1, gate 2).

I found great advice to whoever desires to go through the journey of trying to detoxify their character and become a more refined creation in a letter which was written by the Ramban (Nahmanides, Spain, 1194-1270, rabbi, kabbalist and physician) to his son and here is its translation:

"Hear, my son, the instruction of your father and don't abandon the teaching of your mother" (Proverbs 1:8). Always speak your words pleasantly to everyone at any time, this way you will be saved from anger, a very undesirable characteristic, which causes people to do wrong. As our Rabbis said: Whoever gets angry all kinds of "gehinom" control him (Nedarim 22a) as it says, "Cast out anger from your heart, and remove evil from your flesh." (Ecclesiastes 12:10) "Evil" here means gehinom, as it says: "...and the wicked are destined for the day of evil" (Proverbs 16:4). Once you have been saved from anger, the quality of humility will enter your heart, which is the best of all the good characteristics, as it says, "Following humility comes the fear of Hashem" (Proverbs 22:4). Through humility fear of Hashem will enter your heart. It will always make you think about from where you came, and to where you are going, and that you are only a maggot and a worm while alive, and the same after death (Avot 3:1). It will remind you before Whom you will be judged, before the King of Glory, as it says: "Even the heaven and the heavens of heaven can't contain You" (Kings I 8:27) "How much less the hearts of people!" (Proverbs 15:11), As it says: "Do I not fill heaven and earth? says Hashem" (Jeremiah 23:24). When you think about all these things, you will have awe of your Creator, and you will be saved from doing wrong and with these characteristics you will be happy with your share. Also, when you will act with humility and be modest before everyone, and have awe of Hashem and of doing wrong, then the spirit of the "Shechina" (divine radiance) and the radiance of its glory will rest upon you, and you will live the life of the World to Come. And now, my son, understand and observe that whoever acts as if he were greater than others is rebelling against the Kingship of Hashem, because he is boasting with the garments of Hashem, as it says: "Hashem reigns, He wears clothes of pride" (Psalms 93:1). And why should one feel proud? If it is because of wealth - "Hashem impoverishes and makes rich…" (Samuel I 2:7). If it is because of honor - it belongs to Hashem, as it says: "And the wealth and the honor come from You" (Divrei Hayamim a) 29:12), and how can a person boast with the honor of his Creator?! And if he is boasting with wisdom, Hashem "takes away the speech of assured men and reasoning from the sages" (Job 12:20): So we see that everyone is the same before Hashem, since with His fury He lowers the proud and when He wishes He raises the low, so lower yourself and Hashem will lift you up.

Therefore, I will now explain to you how to always behave with humility: all your words should be spoken pleasantly, your head bowed, your eyes looking down to the ground and your heart focusing on Hashem, you should not look at the face of the person while speaking with him, consider everyone as greater than yourself. If he is wise or rich, you should respect him and if he is poor and you are richer or wiser than him, think in your heart that you are guiltier than he is, and that he is more worthy than you, because if he does wrong it is through error, while yours is deliberate. In all your speech, actions and thoughts and at every moment think in your heart like you are standing before Hashem, and His Shechinah is above you, for His glory fills the whole world. Speak with fear and awe, as a servant standing before his master, be modest in front of everyone, if someone calls you, don't answer loudly, but pleasantly, as one who stands before his teacher. Be careful to read the Torah all the time so you will be able to fulfill it. When you arise from your learning search what you have learned, if there is something in it that you can put into practice, examine your actions in the morning and evening, this way all your days will be spent in teshuvah (returning to Hashem).

Remove all worldly concerns from your heart at the time of prayer, prepare your heart before Hashem, blessed be He, purify your thoughts and you should think about what you are going to say before you take it out of your mouth, and so should you do all the days of your life in each and everything, this way you won't come to do wrong. This way your speech, actions and thoughts will be honest, your prayer will be pure, clear and clean, directed and accepted before Hashem, blessed be He, as it says: "When their heart is directed to You, listen to them" (Psalms 10:17).

Read this letter at least once a week, in order to fulfill it, walk in its path following Hashem, blessed be He, so that you will succeed in all your ways, and you will merit the World to Come, which is hidden away for the righteous. Every day that you will read this letter, you will be answered from Heaven for whatever will come upon your heart to ask for forever. Amen, Sela" (Igeret haRamban – The Ramban's letter.)

"It is an extremely good deed to be happy all the time and to overcome and push away sadness and depression with all his might. All sicknesses which come upon a person come from lack of happiness…And also the wisest of doctors spoke about it in length - that all sickness comes from depression and sadness, and that joy is a great healing method…And the rule is that he needs to greatly overcome sadness with all his strength and to always be happy, because the nature of a person is to drag himself into depression and sadness because of damages of time, what he has gone through in life and every person has sorrow. That's why he needs to force himself with all his might to always be in a state of happiness and to make himself happy in whatever ways he can, even with silly words"(Likutei Mohoran, part 2:25).   Although it says, "Serve Hashem with gladness, come before Him with joyous song" (Psalms 100:2) we need to remember that it says as well, "Serve Hashem with awe that you may rejoice when there is trembling" (Psalms 2:11).

"…A person needs to strive with all his might to revitalize himself and to see, search and find in himself "positive points" and positive qualities, in order not to get to despair. To rejoice in all the good actions he has merited doing in his life, to turn all the grief, sorrow and sighs into joy and happiness. To make it into a habit, every once in a while, to sing some kind of joyous melody, especially on Shabbat, holidays and days of joy, in order to be happy from night to morning and to increase in songs of joy, since the major way to come close to Hashem, especially for the ones who are distant, is through the aspect of happiness" (Likutei Halachot, Even Haezer Pirya veRivya, Ishut Halacha 3).

"…When a person searches and sees that he is distant from his Creator, and he is full of regrets and shortcomings and it seems to him that he is distant from goodness, that's exactly the time to search, ask and find in himself some goodness, since it's impossible that he has never done any positive deed in his life. Even if the little goodness that he has done is full of stains (since it wasn't pure goodness and was mixed with some negativity), it's not possible that he doesn't have at least one "positive point" and so he shall keep searching and finding in himself more and more positive deeds. And so he will keep doing, and finding in himself more and more positive points. By judging himself for good and finding more and more positive points, even though he might have done some negative, he can truly get himself out of "debt" and into "credit". Then he can merit to walk the right path and that's the aspect of "just a little longer and you will see there will be no wicked one" (Psalms 37:10). By the "just a little longer" searching for more and more positive points, "there will be no wicked one".

This will bring him to become more positive and happier and then he'll be able to turn and talk to his Creator by the "just a little longer" (positive points) that he finds in himself. Then he can thank and sing to his Creator. By doing so we separate the positive spirit from the negative and great melodies are created…In the same way, we need to behave towards others (even if they are completely wicked) and find within them positive points." By doing so -"just a little longer and you will see there will be no wicked one"… (Likutei Halachot, Orach Chaim, Hashkamat haBoker 1:1). "When a man will look in the depths of his understanding and will picture in his mind how he comes into being from "ayin" (out of nothing) at every single moment, how can he entertain the thought that he is suffering, or has any hardships related to "children, life and livelihood," or whatever other worldly sufferings? For the "ayin" which is Creator's Wisdom is the source of life, goodness and delight. It is the "Eden" (paradise) that is beyond the World to Come, except that, because it is not apprehensible, one imagines that he is suffering, or afflicted. In truth, however, "No evil descends from above," and everything is good, though it is not apprehended, because of its greatness and abundant goodness. And this is the essence of the faith for which man was created: to believe that "There is no place without the Creator" and "In the light of the King's Face there is life." Accordingly, "Strength and joy are wherever He is," because He is only good all the time. And that's why before everything, a person should be happy and joyous every single moment and truly live by his faith in the Creator, Who gives him life and goodness at every moment" (Igeret haKodesh 11). As the famous saying goes: "Think good and it will be good" (Tzemach Tzedek).

25

Speech Detox

It's a well known thing how important it is to control the words coming out of our mouth. Although it seems like an obvious and easy thing to do, many times we tend to forget and underestimate its value and importance. We all need reminders and tricks in order to become better at practicing it. There is a story that I heard once about a kid that used to be "sharp tongued". He didn't believe in guarding his mouth or in the power and effect of using bad language. Every time he used to get upset or angry, his mouth started pouring out all the "precious" words which cannot be found in the dictionary. His father was concerned and didn't know what to do about it. One day, when his son was bad mouthing out loud, an idea came to his head. "Come with me", he said to his son. "Let me show you something. I want you to do me a favor. You see this piece of wood. Every time you get upset or angry I want you to take a hammer and a nail and knock the nail into the wood. The angrier you are, the harder you should hit." "But why?" said his son, "and for how long?" "Don't worry," said his father, "Just for a week or two. I just want to show you something". And so it was. Every time the son had a temper tantrum, he ran to the back yard, grabbed the hammer and knocked the nail in as hard as he could. After a week, his father asked him to come with him to the back yard again.

"Show me the wood you used," he said. "How was it to knock those nails down? Did you like it?" "Of course I did," said the son. "It was a great relief and I felt much better after. Why do you ask?" "I'll let you know in a minute," said the father, "but first, here is a pair of pliers. Try to take those nails out."

His son started pulling them out. He could not believe how much strength, time and sweat he needed to do so. After a while he proudly said to his father, "I'm done dad. What next?"

"How was it?" said his father.

"Really hard."

"Was it easier or harder than knocking them in?" asked his father.

"It was much harder, nothing to compare."

"You see son, that's how it is when you hurt people with words. It's very easy to shoot it out but it's very hard and sometimes impossible to take it back."

The son was shocked and a little tear rolled down his

cheek. "I guess the holes in the wood will also stay there forever…"

King David says, "Who is the man who desires life, who loves days of seeing good? Guard your tongue from evil, and your lips from speaking deceit" (Psalms 34:13-14). King Solomon who was wiser than any other man says, "One who guards his mouth and his tongue guards his soul from troubles" (Proverbs 21:23).

He also says, "Death and life are in the power of the tongue…" (Proverbs 18:21). Rabban Shimon the son Gamliel says, "All my days I grew up among the Sages and did not find anything better for one's person then silence…" (Avot 1:17).

"A person earns for each and every moment he closes his mouth, the hidden light that no angel or creation can imagine" (Midrash). A way to exercise paying attention to what we say and to speak less can be done by trying to be silent for an hour and then for two and then for a day or two and so on. You can use a notepad and a pen whenever you must "say" something. It's helpful to try it on days when you don't need to communicate very much with people or maybe at night or on Shabbat and weekends. A great idea that can be fun for the whole family is to play the "quiet game" with or without prizes. Slowly you'll begin to realize that you pay much more attention to what comes out of your mouth. "He who guards his mouth and tongue merits being enclothed with the Divine spirit" (Zohar Parshat Chukat).

"He should make fences for himself, staying away from a crowd, not to talk about any person, and with whoever he slipped with his tongue and spoke badly about, he should go and make peace and then guard his mouth for the rest of his life even more, so that his speech will only be in words of holiness and Torah, other than what he needs and for his livelihood. Then he will be able to say about himself "lucky are our old days which overcame the regrets of our young days" (Shmirat Halashon, part 2, Parshat Ki Tavo).

Although guarding the tongue is a huge achievement, we need to remember to watch everything we see, hear, speak, eat, breathe, think and experience since they all have a great effect on who we are. After all we are what we see, what we hear, speak, eat, etc. The question is what can be done with damaging words that were thrown upon us with the years, like "You will never be..." or "You are so..." etc. or with a poor self-image? There is an idea in Jewish law that "Kmo shekolet, kacha polet" meaning to make something that is impure pure again, the impurity needs to be removed the way it entered. Since it's impossible to locate all the people that made those negative statements, and to ask them to say the opposite, we can do it ourselves by putting down on paper positive phrases of things we feel we are lacking or want to change about ourselves and our lives and saying them out loud a few times a day. The more we say them, the quicker the negativity will be removed and positivity will take its place. The next step is to close our eyes and imagine ourselves in the place we want to be. This imaginary exercise should also be done as often as possible. This way we will have a better chance to be in the reality we're after.

26

The Power Within

Changing our personal world and the world in general starts with the way we think, which affects the way feel, which affects the way we speak, which affects the way we act, which affects our personality, which affects the way life treats us, which affects the way the world is...

Speech is so powerful that it is a Godly commandment for the "kohanim" (the children of Aaron) to bless the children of Israel: "Hashem spoke to Moses saying: Speak to Aaron and his sons, saying: This is how you shall bless the children of Israel, saying to them: May Hashem bless you and watch over you. May Hashem cause His countenance to shine to you and favor you. May Hashem raise His countenance toward you and grant you peace, and they shall bestow My Name upon the children of Israel, so that I will bless them" (Numbers 6:22-27). More than that, if the service of the "kohanim" (priests) was done without the correct intension or speech it could invalidate the entire service. Isn't that amazing how much power our thoughts and words have but still we forget so many times to practice thinking and speaking in a positive and kind way. Imagine what the world would be like if we practiced this fundamental idea.

Being kind and thankful from within, which means to see, feel, believe, admit and say it on regular basis every day as many times as we can is a very powerful tool to make the change to a positive vibe. Think about it, what kind of people you like to be around, kind or inconsiderate and mean; thankful or critical; smiling or frowning; generous or stingy? Just like we are attracted to positive people, positivity and abundance are attracted to them as well. Many times we can use the help of our feelings to indicate where we need to change our thoughts and our focus. If we feel good, we are usually on the right track. If we feel bad it means we need to change our thoughts and our focus. It's very hard and probably impossible to think a good thought and to feel bad.

Our life is a mirror of what we feel inside, and our feelings are usually in our control. Our thoughts play a major role in creating our reality. We are creating our reality all the time. So when we don't like our reality, it's a sign that we need to reevaluate our thoughts. If we pay attention carefully, we will realize that we are thinking all the time. Many times we don't realize the negativity of our thoughts, which unconsciously may attract unwanted negativity into our lives. For example, worrying about money can bring about financial issues. When someone worries about money, they are broadcasting their lack of money, which can attract a lack of money. Instead we should recognize the thought and change it to the abundance channel.

Since we are thinking all the time, we are attracting all the time. That's why the more we are aware and in control of our thoughts, we become better at focusing on the things we want in our life, and attract more quickly the reality we are after. Only you can navigate your thoughts. The same applies to speech. Positive words attract the positive, for example, "I can do it". Negative speech attracts the negative, for example, "I don't know" or "I can't do it".

The Creator, Hashem, God, the Universe or whatever you choose to call this magnificent power, is unlimited. It's not our job to figure out how our abundance will come about, but it is our job and responsibility to broadcast our wishes in a positive and precise way. We can practice controlling our thoughts and speech, and even take it to the next level by playing "make believe" or creating a vision board and trying to live the reality we wish for as much as we can. The more senses we utilize and the more we believe and ask, the better we get at it and the faster we attract our abundance. Always remember that all the abundance has already

been created. It's just our job to find a way to attract it. Abundance in all forms such as healing, relationships and material needs to name a few.
Whatever you want to attract from others try to do for others. If you want people to smile to you, try to smile to others. Whatever you want to receive, try to give to others generously and with joy.

27
Soul Remedy

"And He said, If you hearken to the voice of Hashem, your God, and you do what is proper in His eyes, and you listen closely to His commandments and observe all His statutes, all the sicknesses that I have visited upon Egypt I will not visit upon you, for I am Hashem your Healer" (Exodus 15:26). King Solomon says: "…charity will save from death" (Proverbs 10:2). "Charity guards him who is honest in his way…" (Proverbs 13:6). "The ransom of a man's soul is his wealth…" (Proverbs 13:8).

In the Rosh Hashana prayers it says "teshuvah", "tefillah" and "tzedakah" remove the severity of the decree. "Teshuvah" – returning to Hashem, admitting our mistakes in order not to repeat them and or fasting. "Tefillah" – prayer, saying psalms, talking to Hashem and voice. "Tzedakah" – charity, giving of help typically in the form of money.

"TESHUVAH" & FASTING

"It is the remedy for all sickness and afflictions" (Tikunei HaZohar, Tikun 63). The Rambam explains that "teshuvah" is "when a wrongdoer will go away from his mistake, remove it from his thoughts and will resolve in his heart not to do it anymore as it says: "Let the wrongdoer leave his way and the iniquitous man his thoughts" (Isaiah 55:7)" (Rambam Tesuvah 2:2, see for more details).

"Teshuvah" as an act is explained in the prayer books as fasting. Fasting by itself separates between life and death. If a person does not eat or drink they cannot survive. That's why fasting and eating are the connector and the barrier between physicality and spirituality. Spirits do not eat or drink but physical beings must eat and drink. Fasting also has endless healing potential, when it is done properly, since it gives the body the chance to heal itself. I believe that it works similarly with our souls. The less we eat the more spiritual we become and the more we can connect to the Divine. I could easily write an entire book only about fasting. It is a fascinating subject. I believe that watching what we eat and say and trying to eat and talk as little as needed is life changing and can bring a lot of light into our life. Just think about all the weight we can lose and all the regrets we could save by not saying things that we wish we hadn't. The only commandment to fast in the Torah is on "Yom haKipurim" (the day of atonement) from evening to evening, without doing any work, which will serve as atonement. "And Hashem spoke to Moses, saying: But on the tenth of this seventh month, it is a day of atonement, it shall be a holy occasion for you; you shall afflict yourselves…You shall not perform any work on that very day, for it is a day of atonement, for you to gain atonement before Hashem, your God" (Leviticus 23:26-28).

Two more examples of fasting are when Moses fasted for 40 days and nights with no water and no bread when he merited the revelation of the Ten Commandments. The second time he fasted as well for 40 days and nights with no water and no bread was to rectify the entire nation's wrongdoing.

Today there are different opinions and ways how to do so in private. One opinion is dry fasting (without eating or drinking) for each wrong deed. The number of the fast days needed is calculated by taking the number of fast days required for each wrong deed and multiplying this number by the number of times the deed was done (Ari Zal, Shaar Ruach haKodesh, Tikkun 16-22). Another opinion is fasting four times for three days and nights a year: before Rosh Hashana, before Yom Kippur, before 10 Tevet and before 17 Tammuz. Once in a lifetime is enough to nullify the bad decrees that were supposed to come upon him in this world, but not in the world to come (Shaar haKavanot daf 90 amud 2). There is also an opinion that says: "…Redeem your regrets through charity…" (Daniel 4:24) and the way to do it, according to some opinions, is to give charity two thirds times the value of 19.2 grams of pure silver, times the number of fast days needed. In our generation the custom is to increase even beyond that, as much as possible (Igeret haTeshuva, end of ch. 3).

"TEFILLAH" (PRAYER)

This is explained in the prayer book simply as "voice". The Rambam explains it as an action of praising Hashem, making a request of Him, and thanking Him for the abundant goodness that He has granted, every person according to their ability (Rambam Tefillah 1:2). There are five things which disturb one from praying, even though the time for prayer has arrived: 1) the purification of one's hands (i.e. washing the hands in water until the wrist), 2) the covering of nakedness, 3) the purity of the place of prayer (i.e. not to pray in a place of filth, a bathhouse, etc.) 4) things that might bother and distract one (e.g. needing to relieve oneself), 5) the proper intention of one's heart, i.e. clear his mind from all thoughts and envision himself as standing before the Divine Presence (Rambam Tefillah ch. 4).

"Hashem is close to all who call upon Him, to all who call upon Him in truth" (Psalms 145:18). Rabbi Nachman of Breslov (1772-1810, Ukraine, great grandson of the Baal Shem Tov, the founder of the Hassidic movement) talks about "Hitbodedut" (self seclusion) and explains that "hitbodedut" is an extremely high level and it means to set for himself an hour or more to seclude himself in some sort of room or field and to speak in detail to his Creator about whatever is in his heart, to humbly request from Hashem blessed be He to bring him closer to serve Him truly. This prayer and conversation will be in his native language…and he will talk to Hashem about whatever is in his heart, his regrets about the past and humbly request to truly come close to Him from now on, etc. everyone according to where he is at. And he will try very hard to accustom himself to do so on a daily basis at a set hour and the rest of the day he should be happy.

This is a very precious custom and a great way and advice to come close to Him blessed be He. This general advice includes everything in it since whatever he is lacking in serving Hashem, or if he is completely distant from serving Him, he should speak to Him about everything and ask Him for anything.

Even if sometimes he feels blocked and cannot open his mouth and speak in front Him at all, this in itself is a good thing. The good thing is that he desires and is preparing himself to speak, only he can't. It's good advice to create his own conversation and prayer from this situation and scream out loud asking for Hashem's mercy for being so distant that he can't even speak. To help him and have mercy on him to open his mouth so he can speak in front of Him. You should know that some of the greatest righteous people explained that they reached their level only by using this method. The wise ones will understand the greatness of this method which can lift a person higher and higher and is available to everyone no matter where they are holding. By doing so they can reach high levels. Lucky is the one that will hold tightly to this advice (Likutei Mohoran part 2:25).

"…by secluding himself and speaking to his Creator he merits to nullify all the lusts and undesirable characteristics, to the level of completely nullifying his physicality and including himself in his Source. The best time for "hitbodedut" is at night, the time that the world is free from mundane concerns, since in the daytime the majority of people run after this physical world and this disturbs and confuses a person from cleaving and including himself within Hashem. It is best for "hitbodedut" to be in a special place, such as outside the city on a private route, a place where people don't usually go. The reason is, since a place where people usually go to during the daytime, disturbs the "hitbodedut" and makes it impossible for the person to nullify and include himself within Hashem, even though these people who are busy with the physical world are not there at the moment. That's why he should walk by himself at night on a private route in a place that nobody is there and seclude himself and turn his heart and mind away from all worldly matters and nullify everything until he merits the aspect of true nullification…"(Likutei Mohoran, part 1:52).

Rabbi Nachman said if a person merited to hear the praises and singing of the weeds, how each weed sings praises to the Creator... and how beautiful and pleasant it is to hear their singing, he will understand why it is great to serve Hashem in awe among them...and to be secluded in the field among the plants and truly pour his heart before Hashem.

He also said that "Hitbodedut" is best done outside of the city in a place of wild plants because they help with the awakening of the heart (Hishtapchut haNefesh 28). Even though ideally "Hitbodedut" is best done in nature, there are other options as well. The most important thing is the actual conversation, not the location. "It's very good for a person to have a special room for himself to serve Hashem there, especially with "hitbodedut" and conversation between himself and his Creator. Even sitting by himself in this special room is very good and if he doesn't have such a room he can find different ways to do "hitbodedut" like under his "talit" (prayer shawl) or under the blanket while he is in bed, like King David used to do, or to pretend that he is reading a book and talk to Hashem.

It's possible to find other tricks, whoever really desires to do so, especially since "hitbodedut" is the greatest since it is the root of holiness and purity, but still it's better to try to have a special room" (Hishtapchut Ha-Nefesh, 39). He said as well that the conversation a person has with his Creator is a new and original route and prayer, said from his heart. For that reason the "accusers" are usually not around to damage it (since they are not familiar with this new and original route or prayer) (Likutei Mohoran, part 2:97). "Hitbodedut" can be a remedy ("segulah") for overcoming regrets. One day a week a person should isolate himself to be with his Creator and connect his thoughts to Him like an arrow to a target. Like he is standing in front of Hashem and speaking to Him gently like a son to his father. According to the capability and strength of a person he should do so one day in fifteen days or once a month, but not less. It can benefit the soul seven times more than learning" (The Book of Haredim, ch. 65, 73). Rabbi Nachman advised his followers to do "hitbodedut" for an hour each day. It is a commandment from the Torah, once a day at whatever hour he wants, to beg as much as he can and ask for his needs in a pure, clean way (The Book of Haredim 38:11).

TEHILLIM (PSALMS)

"Hashem, my God, I cried out to you and you healed me" (Psalms 30:3). Most of the book of Psalms is attributed to King David. It is believed that it was written through Divine inspiration and that reading it on a regular basis can bring a person to have a taste of this inspiration. It contains 150 psalms (the same number as the numerical value of the Hebrew word to redeem, "pidyon"). They are divided into 5 books, parallel to the five books of Moses. There is a custom to finish the book once a month, by reading the daily portion, or once a week reading a set portion each day. This is done by using the markings inside the book. Some have the custom to say the entire book on special days of the year. Obviously these are only tips for people who are looking for a systematic way to say psalms on a regular basis and everyone can say as many psalms as they want, whenever they want. It's best to say them from midnight to sunset the following day.

Although some psalms mention a great deal of hardship and request tests and challenges, the book of psalms is believed to be a spiritual healing tool, to the level that a whole book was written explaining the remedies of each of the 150 psalms. ("Shimush Tehillim", attributed to Rav Hai haGaon, 939-1038, Babylonia.) However, it is important to remember that the purpose of saying psalms is to wake up the soul and to cleave to the Creator, which is the true remedy for everything and not to make the mistake of saying psalms with the intention that the actual words are healing (see Mishneh Torah Avoda Zara 11:12).

This is also the reason why it is so important to say the "yehi ratzon" prayer before saying psalms. By saying it we are meditating to say psalms with the right intention. Some say that it is best to read them in a way that you identify with what is happening in the psalm, to the level that you are living the plot, understand the words and are saying them out loud with excitement and with a melody. The next level is to say the words quietly. There are some opinions that say it is enough just to move the lips when saying psalms. The idea is try to say them as close as possible to the way King

David said them. That's also why some explain that when we say in the Rosh Hashana prayer book that "regret, prayer and charity remove the severity of the decree", the word "prayer" refers to saying psalms, because by saying the prayers of King David, his merit will protect us on this day.

Here are four out of the endless sayings and praises about the greatness of the book of psalms and saying its verses: "We have nothing greater than the book of psalms which includes everything. And the one who says psalms is like praying and learning Torah" (Shalah). "Psalms are keys which fit all the chambers of mercy, healing, salvation and livelihood" (Noam Elimelech). "The one who reads psalms everyday and takes the words out of his mouth and also the one who says the blessing after eating bread out loud, his days and years are prolonged (Rabbi Chaim Falaji). "The one who is accustomed to saying Psalms pushes away calamity and harm from himself, his family and his generation and brings upon them many different kinds of flow of blessings and success" (Emek haMelech p. 15). "These ten chapters of Psalms are miraculous, precious and extremely helpful...I am very strong in all my words but in this I am extremely strong that these ten chapters of Psalms are extremely helpful...16, 32, 41, 42, 59, 77, 90, 105, 137, 150, to be said in this order...It is the "general correction" of all regrets" (Rabbi Nachman of Breslev, Sichot haRan 141).

"If you only knew", the Tzemach Tzedek said, "the

power of verses of Tehillim and their effect in the highest Heavens, you would recite them constantly. Know that the chapters of Tehillim shatter all barriers, they ascend higher and still higher with no interference; they prostrate themselves in supplication before the Master of all worlds, and they effect and accomplish with kindness and compassion" (Hayom Yom 24 Shvat).

We always need to be aware of what we are saying, as words can have a great impact on our life. The same applies to reading. The value of the Book of Psalms is undisputed but we still need to be aware of the words we are saying, especially when reading the psalms where the poet asks Hashem to be tested such as, "Examine me, Hashem, and test me; scrutinize my intellect and my heart" (Psalms 26:2), "Examine me, O Hashem, and know my heart; test me, and know my thoughts" (Psalms 139:23). It is explained that one of the reasons that the story of King David and Bath-sheba happened was because of his request to be tested (Samuel II 11:1). Rabbi Akiva said: "The entire universe is unworthy of the day on which the Song of Songs was given to Israel. All the Writings are holy, but the Song of Songs is the holy of holies" (Midrash Rabbah 1:11).

The "Yehi Ratzon" prayer: "May it be the will before You, Hashem, our God, and the God of our forefathers, Who chose David His servant and his offspring after him, and Who chose songs and praises - that you attend with mercy to the saying of psalms, that I shall say them as if they were recited by King David, of blessed memory, himself, may his merit be a shield over us. And this merit should stand in our favor together with the merit of the verses of the psalms together with the merit of their words and their letters and their vowels and their cantillation notes, and together with the Holy Names that are formed from them, from the initial letters of the words and from the final letters of the words, may their merit serve to bring atonement for our regrets and to cut down tyrants, and cut all the thorns and briars which surround the Supreme Rose, and to unite the Bride of Youth with her Beloved in love, brotherhood, and companionship. And from that unification may there be drawn to us an abundant blessing to our spirit and soul, to purify, forgive and atone our regrets, just as You forgave David who recited these very same psalms before You, as it is said: "Hashem also has forgiven your wrongdoings, you shall not die". May you not take us from this world before our time, until the completion of our years, in a manner that we be able to rectify anything that we need to fix.

May the merit of King David, of blessed memory, shield over us and for us; that You will be patient until we return to You with complete regret. From your treasury of unconditional gifts, be gracious to us - as it is written: "I am compassionate to those whom I favor, and I am merciful to those upon whom I have mercy". And just as we recite before You a song in this world, so let us merit to recite before You - O Hashem, our God - songs and praises in the World to Come. And through the recitation of the psalms arouse the Rose of Sharon to sing with a pleasant voice, with ecstasy and joy. May the glory of the Levanon be given to her, majesty and splendor in the House of our God, speedily in our days. Amen. Selah! Come! Let us sing joyfully to Hashem, let us call out to the Rock of our salvation, Let us greet Him with thanksgiving, with praiseful songs let us call out to Him. For a great God is Hashem, and a great King above all heavenly powers."

28

Psalm Quotes

"A psalm by David. Hashem is my shepherd, I shall lack nothing. He lays me down in green pastures; He leads me beside still waters. He revives my soul; He directs me in paths of righteousness for the sake of His Name. Though I walk in the valley of the shadow of death, I will fear no evil, for You are with me; Your rod and Your staff-they will comfort me. You will prepare a table for me before my enemies; You have anointed my head with oil; my cup is full. Only goodness and kindness shall follow me all the days of my life, and I shall dwell in the House of Hashem for many long years" (Psalm 23).

"Who may ascend the mountain of Hashem, and who may stand in His holy place? He who has clean hands and a pure heart, who has not used My Name in vain or sworn falsely. He shall receive a blessing from Hashem, and kindness from God, his deliverer" (Psalms 24:3-5). "Hashem, my God, I cried out to You, and You healed me" (Psalms 30:3).

"Exalt Hashem with me, and let us extol His Name together. I sought Hashem and He answered me; He delivered me from all my fears. Those who look to Him are radiant; their faces are never humiliated. This poor man called, and Hashem heard; He delivered him from all his tribulations. The angel of Hashem camps around those who fear Him, and rescues them. Taste and see that Hashem is good; fortunate is the man who trusts in Him. Fear Hashem, you His holy ones, for those who fear Him suffer no want. Young lions may want and hunger, but those who seek Hashem shall not lack any good thing. Come, children, listen to me; I will teach you the fear of Hashem. Who is the man who desires life, who loves long life wherein to see goodness? Guard your tongue from evil, and your lips from speaking deceit. Turn away from evil and do good, seek peace and pursue it. The eyes of Hashem are directed toward the righteous, and His ears toward their cry. The wrath of Hashem is upon the evildoers, to excise their memory from the earth. But when they cry out, Hashem hears, and saves them from all their troubles. Hashem is close to the broken-hearted, and saves those with a crushed spirit. Many are the afflictions of a righteous person, but Hashem rescues him from them all. He protects all his bones; not one of them is broken. Evil brings death upon the wicked, and the enemies of the righteous are condemned. Hashem redeems the soul of His servants; all who take shelter in Him are not condemned" (Psalms 34:4-23).

"Hashem, Your kindness is in the heavens; Your faithfulness is till the skies. Your righteousness is like the mighty mountains, Your judgments are like the vast deep waters; man and beast You save, Hashem. How precious is Your kindness, O God; man takes shelter in the shadow of Your wings. They will be filled by the abundance of Your house; from the stream of Your Eden, You will give them to drink. For the source of life is with You; in Your Light do we see light. Extend Your kindness to those who know You, and Your righteousness to the upright of heart" (Psalms 36:6-11).

"Trust in Hashem and do good; then will you abide in the land and be nourished by faith. Delight in Hashem, and He will grant you the desires of your heart. Cast your needs upon Hashem; rely on Him, and He will take care…Hashem appreciates the days of the innocent; their inheritance will last forever. They will not be shamed in times of calamity, and in days of famine they will be satisfied… I have been a youth, I have also aged; yet I have not seen the righteous forsaken, nor his offspring begging bread. All day he is kind and lends; his offspring are a blessing. Turn away from evil and do good, and you will dwell forever. For Hashem loves justice, he will not abandon his pious ones-they are protected forever; but the offspring of the wicked are cut off. The righteous shall inherit the earth and dwell upon it forever…Watch the innocent, and observe the upright, for the future of such a man is peace…" (Psalm 37).

"Indeed, You desire truth in the innermost parts; teach me the wisdom of concealed things. Purge me with hyssop and I shall be pure; cleanse me and I shall be whiter than snow. Let me hear joy and gladness; then the bones which You have shattered will rejoice. Hide Your face from my wrongdoings, and erase all my trespasses. Create in me a pure heart, O God, and renew within me an upright spirit. Do not cast me out of Your presence, and do not take Your Spirit of Holiness away from me. Restore to me the joy of Your deliverance, and uphold me with a spirit of generosity... For You do not desire that I bring sacrifices, nor do You wish burnt offerings. The offering to God is a contrite spirit; a contrite and broken heart, God, You do not disdain…" (Psalm 51).

"Cast your burden upon Hashem, and He will sustain you; He will never let the righteous man falter. And You, O God, will bring them down to the nethermost pit; bloodthirsty and treacherous men shall not live out half their days; but I will trust in You" (Psalms 55:23-24).

"To God alone does my soul hope, for my hope is from Him. He alone is my rock and salvation, my stronghold; I shall not falter. My salvation and honor is upon God; the rock of my strength-my refuge is in God. Trust in Him at all times, O nation, pour out your hearts before Him; God is a refuge for us forever" (Psalms 62:6-9).

"Come listen, all you who fear God, and I will relate what He has done for my soul. I called to Him with my mouth, with exaltation beneath my tongue. Had I seen iniquity in my heart, Hashem would not have listened. But in truth, God heard; He gave ear to the voice of my prayer. Blessed is God Who has not turned away my prayer or His kindness from me" (Psalms 66:16-20).

"You who dwells in the shelter of the Most High, who abides in the shadow of the Omnipotent: I say of Hashem who is my refuge and my stronghold, my God in whom I trust, that He will save you from the ensnaring trap, from the destructive pestilence. He will cover you with His wings and you will find refuge under His wings; His truth is a shield and an armor. You will not fear the terror of the night, nor the arrow that flies by day; the pestilence that prowls in the darkness, nor the destruction that ravages at noon. A thousand may fall at your side, and ten thousand at your right, but it shall not reach you. You need only look with your eyes, and you will see the retribution of the wicked. Because You Hashem are my shelter, and You have made the Most High your haven, no evil will befall you, no plague will come near your tent. For He will instruct His angels on your behalf, to guard you in all your ways. They will carry you in their hands, lest you injure your foot upon a rock. You will tread upon the lion and the viper; you will trample upon the young lion and the serpent. Because he desires Me, I will deliver him; I will fortify him, for he knows My Name. When he calls on Me, I will answer him; I am with him in distress. I will deliver him and honor him. I will satiate him with long life, and show him My deliverance" (Psalm 91).

"My soul, bless Hashem; forget not all His favors: Who forgives all your sins, Who heals all your illnesses; Who redeems your life from the grave, Who crowns you with kindness and mercy; Who satisfies your mouth with goodness; like the eagle, your youth is renewed. Hashem executes righteousness and justice for all the oppressed" (Psalms 103:2-6).

"The beginning of wisdom is fear of Hashem; sound wisdom for all who practice it-his praise endures forever" (Psalms 111:10).

"Praise Hashem! Fortunate is the man who fears Hashem, and desires His commandments intensely. His descendants will be mighty on the earth; he will be blessed with an upright generation. Wealth and riches are in his house, and his righteousness endures forever. Even in darkness light shines for the upright, Compassionate, Merciful, and Just. Good is the man who is compassionate and lends, provides for his own needs with discretion. For he will never falter; the righteous man will be an eternal remembrance. He will not be afraid of a bad tiding; his heart is steadfast, secure in Hashem. His heart is steadfast, he does not fear, until he sees his oppressors. He has distributed, giving to the needy. His righteousness will endure forever; his might will be uplifted in honor" (Psalms 112:1-9).

"A song of ascents. Fortunate is every man who fears Hashem, who walks in His ways. When you eat of the labor of your hands, you will be happy, and you will have goodness. Your wife will be like a fruitful vine in the inner chambers of your house; your children will be like olive saplings around your table. Behold, so will be blessed the man who fears Hashem. May Hashem bless you out of Zion, and may you see the goodness of Jerusalem all the days of your life. And may you see children to your children; peace upon Israel" (Psalm 128).

29

Tzedakah

"Tzedakah" (charity) is explained in the prayer book simply as "money". Here are some ideas on how to give charity more consciously: "A poor person should be given according to what he lacks. If he doesn't have clothing, we clothe him. If he doesn't have house wares, we buy him house wares. If he doesn't have a wife, we marry him to a woman. If it is a woman, we marry her to a man. Even if a poor man used to ride a horse and have a helper run in front of him, and the poor person lost his possessions, we buy him a horse to ride on and a helper to run in front of him, as it says: "…whatever is lacking to him" (Deuteronomy 15:8). You should give him what he is lacking but you do not need to make him rich" (Rambam Matanot Aniyim 7:1-2). And if there is more than one poor person, who should we give to first? A poor person who is his relative comes before anyone else. The poor of his home come before the poor of his city. The poor of his city come before the poor of another city as it says: "…to your brother, to your poor, and to your destitute in your Land (Deuteronomy 15:11)" (Rambam Matanot Aniyim 7:13).

There are eight levels in charity one higher than the next: The highest is to give a person a gift, a loan, a partnership or to find him a job so he would not get to the point of needing help. The next level is to give to the poor in a way that he wouldn't know who he gave to and the poor wouldn't know who gave to him. Similar to this is to put money into a charity box, on condition that he knows that the one in charge is wise and loyal. The next level is that he will know who he is giving to but the poor wouldn't know. It is better to do this if a person doesn't know that the one in charge of the charity box is wise and loyal. The next level is that the poor person will know who gave it to him but the one who gave wouldn't know who he gave it to. The next level is to give him in his hand before he asks for it. The next level is to give it to him after he asks. The next level is that he will give less that he is supposed to but he will do it in a pleasant way. The lowest level is to give with sadness (Rambam Matanot Aniyim 10:7-14). "The amount of giving if a person can, is according to the needs of the poor and if he can't, the best is to give a fifth of his income and if he can't he should give at least a tenth of his income" (Shulchan Aruch, Yoreh

Deah, Tzedakah, 249:1). Rabbi Shneur Zalman of Liadi (1745-1812, first Rebbe of Chabad) explains "Now the essence of regret is in the heart, for through regret from the depth of the heart one arouses the depth, i.e., the ultimate degree of this Supreme light. But in order for this light to continue to illuminate in the higher and lower worlds, there must be an actual arousal from below in the form of action, i.e., the practice of charity and kindness without limit and measure.

For just as a man gives out great kindness, in other words, "he pities him who doesn't have" implying that he gives out of his kindness to the utterly destitute individual who does not have anything of his own, without setting a limit or measure to his giving — so, too, the Holy One, blessed be He, gives out His light and goodness in the aspect of the supreme kindness, known as "great kindness", that illuminates infinitely, without limit or measure, within the upper and lower worlds which are all in the aspect of "nothing" in relation to Him, blessed be He, inasmuch as they have nothing at all of their own, and all before Him are considered as nothing. Therefore all the blemishes that a man caused above, in the upper and the lower worlds, through his regrets, are corrected in this way through the act of charity. And this is the meaning of the verse, "God prefers charity and justice over offerings" (Proverbs 21:2), because the sacrifices are defined in terms of quantity, dimension and limitation, while charity can be given out without limit, for the purpose of correcting one's regrets. As for the ruling that "He who gives his money generously should not exceed more than one fifth of his earnings," this applies only to one who has not done wrong, or who has corrected his regrets…, as indeed all the blemishes Above should be corrected. But as to him who still needs to heal his soul, the healing of his soul is obviously just as important as the healing of his body, where money does not count in other words, when someone is physically sick he wouldn't think twice how much to spend in order to be cured, so too with the healing of his soul. As it says: "Whatever a man has he would give up for his soul" (Job 2:4) (Igeret HaKodesh, Ch. 10).

The Rambam (Matanot Aniyim 10:2) writes "No-one will ever become poor from giving charity and nothing bad or any damage will ever be caused by it. As it says: "The product of charity shall be peace" (Isaiah 32:17). And whoever is merciful, there will be mercy upon him as it says: "…and He will give you mercy and be merciful to you…" (Deuteronomy 13:18). Some people try to practice the essence of the idea of what it says in the New Year (Rosh Hashana) prayers that "teshuvah", "tefillah" and "tzedakah" remove the severity of the decree" on a daily basis. They do so by trying not to eat or drink from dawn until after prayer, which represents the aspect of fasting, giving a few coins to charity before prayer, which represents the aspect of charity and actual prayer.

30

We Have What We Need

We are told over and over again how important it is to be happy. "Laughter is the best medicine" is a saying that all of us are familiar with. But how many of us are truly happy from within? How many of us genuinely feel rich and blessed? "Who is rich? He who is happy with his lot" (Avot 4:1). We've all heard this famous teaching of our Sages but how on earth can we put it into practice? This is something that has been on my mind for a long time. If I stop for a moment and look at life, I honestly believe that Hashem gives everyone everything they need and much more. Even when things seem like they're not working, may times it's a road sign directing us to a better place. The trick is to realize it and recognize all the times that Hashem is sending us exactly what we need. It might not come at exactly the time we wanted it or in the exact package we were expecting, but it is exactly what we needed and exactly the way that we should receive it. Not everything we want is the best for us and we can't always see the full picture. Our society is so used to getting everything "right at this time" but not necessarily at the right time. It seems to be human nature that whatever we have we want double. "One who has one hundred wants two hundred" (Kohelet Rabbah 1:34). That's why many times when someone doesn't have very much they don't want too much. Of course we were created with this character for a reason. It is an excellent tool for self improvement and doing good deeds. However, if it is used in an inappropriate, materialistic context, it can lead a person to always feel that they don't have enough and that whatever they think they are lacking is the missing key to their doorway to happiness.

People also have a tendency to look at what others have and define their dreams and goals according to that. Such a person could live their entire life without a single moment of happiness, always feeling that something is missing in their life, since they always want what they don't have, even though they might have everything. "Do not desire the table of kings, for your table is greater than theirs..." (Avot 6:5).

Your reality is what you make it. When I was a child, I always wanted to travel. In our kitchen we had a sink with a very unusual faucet that for whatever the reason reminded me of a boat. I would close the kitchen door and stand next to the sink and in my mind I was really in the kitchen of a cruise ship. That was my reality for that moment. It's not that I didn't want to be where I was. In my mind I was exactly where I wanted to be. I chose to see my reality in a way that made me feel good.

In Tales of Ancient Times, Rabbi Nachman of Breslev tells the story of the Clever One and the Simple One. The Clever One was very bright and the Simple One was simple-minded and naive, not foolish, only his intellect was unsophisticated. The Clever One was always dissatisfied with his life, thinking that his happiness was to be found somewhere else, either in a different country or by gaining more wisdom.

The Simple One on the other hand was always very happy. He had all the kinds of food, drink and clothing he wanted, even though he was very poor. For example, when he was hungry, he would ask his wife to bring him something to eat. She would bring him bread and water. After this he would ask for beans and sauce. Again she would bring him bread and water. He would praise the food "How delicious was that sauce". In truth he really tasted in the bread the taste of the food he wanted because of his simplicity, great happiness and state of mind. And so it was with drinks and clothing.

The Clever One suffered all his life, learning many professions to ensure that he always had "something to fall back on". He couldn't relate to others because of his sophisticated way of thinking and the knowledge he had gained through his continuous travel and study. He was in agony over any mistake he made in his constant pursuit of perfection.

The Simple One became one of the king's governors, as the king sought out a simple man who would govern the state with truth and uprightness. A change of fortune brings wisdom and the Simple One gained more understanding. He ruled with simplicity, as he was accustomed and led the country with truth and uprightness, without a trace of corruption. What's interesting is that he was able to reach the level of the Clever One but the Clever One could not come to the level of the Simple One.

We are all guests in the Creator's international park. It's just a question of what we choose to do here. It's our right to be healthy, to come close to the Creator and learn and enjoy His Creation. Hashem has given us free treasures that every single person can access at any time. "The best things in life are free". Being silent, talking to Hashem, saying Psalms, exercising, sleeping, laughing, being with our loved ones, etc.

Most people can make the choice of buying healthy food, putting a water filter on their faucet and drinking clean water, getting eight hours of sleep, using clean sheets, having a hot shower, a warm meal, talking to their friends, going to the park, buying a new shirt, going for a walk, exercising and the list goes on. You see, Western society is mostly a materialistically rich society, but for whatever the reason, we take everything for granted and dream of long and expensive vacations, meeting new people and being around new people. We always dream about what we don't have, when we have so much abundance around us. We can use the heater, the air conditioner; we can be warm or cool whenever we want. We are such a rich society, but still so many feel that they are poor.

While many of the "successful" and "rich" people many times lack family, lack friends, lack going to the park and getting a fresh, brisk walk and spending quality time with their loved ones, they live in a house that looks like a palace but it's "cold" like a freezer. They probably never walked bare foot in their back yard if they ever walked there at all. And if you talk to them they'll probably tell you that they don't feel successful and they hope that next year they'll make more money and that the whole family thing can wait. "First I want to get a bigger house and a better position at work and hopefully another zero on my paycheck".

It might be hard to change this state of mind, but it's definitely possible and it's definitely necessary in order not to get to self-destruction. It can take a month, a year or ten years. It doesn't matter but we have to get on that route. This is the only way to be alive. All we have is the present, nothing else. It has always been like that and probably always will be.

It's not that being wealthy is a bad thing. It's the blind race after these never-ending physical and materialistic goals, without living our life. After all, all we take with us when we leave this international park are our good deeds. By not wanting what we don't have, and appreciating what we do, we understand that happiness is not a state of location or possessions; it's a state of mind. And many times when we don't get what we want it's because we don't really want it or we don't really need it and actually many possessions can mean many worries.

In summary, most of the time, most of us if not all of us have everything. We just need to learn to open our eyes and identify it. This is the way to the real wealth which is available to all of us.

31

Illumination

The Baal Shem Tov once said, "Everything is by Divine Providence. If a leaf is turned over by a breeze, it is only because this has been specifically ordained by the Creator to serve a particular function within the purpose of creation". Each and every organism has a place and a role on the planet. The trick is to find ours. When we discover it, act on it and live according to the "teachings" of the Universe we might be able to reach illumination. So what is true illumination?

All the time we receive messages. We need to be like a wheel, to be in motion all the time. Whatever comes from above, whatever messages or knowledge we receive, we take and give to others. Different people say this idea in different ways, but the idea is essentially the same. Whatever you receive, you need to give. If you receive "kedusha" (holiness) or illumination and pass it on to others, then you increase light and Godliness in the world. On the other hand, if a person taps into negative energy and then passes that onto others, they increase darkness in the world. For example, if a person grew up in an abusive household and then passes this negativity or darkness onto their family, they increase darkness in the world.

We all have a need to give and if we aren't fulfilling this need then it causes a certain blockage and sometimes the person might not even feel it. For example, Hashem created women in a way that according to nature they have an innate need to give to another creation. She has the ability to give birth and to give milk to her child. She wants to give and if she doesn't give, she has a certain obstruction or blockage or a certain need that is not fulfilled. In a case where a woman for some reason can't have children, she'll feel a need or a drive to take care of children or to be teacher or maybe to take care of animals. It's all about the need to give.

In order to be in a state of illumination, you need to be in full balance. You need to be receiving and giving all the time. The more this is done in a clean and pure way, the cleaner and purer the light. If you are dealing with Holy things, for example, you learn Torah and you teach Torah, you are channel for Godliness. You are a channel for light, you are illuminated. That's the whole idea. When are you illuminated? When you are doing what you are supposed to be doing. How do you know what you are supposed to be doing? You are supposed to be connected to The Source, to Hashem. The source of the soul is under "the chair of Glory". When you are connected to Godliness, you are receiving Godliness, you are giving Godliness, you are a channel for Godliness, and thus you are illuminated. When a person is not doing this, there is certain kind of blockage. The person receives but they don't give. They become spiritually stagnant, which can lead to being physically stagnant, for example feeling stuck or an inability to move forward in life.

When the vessel, the capability to receive is full, the person cannot receive any more light. They can't understand what's wrong with them – they have something to give but they don't give it and this leads to frustration and anger, inner chaos and instability. It can even lead to deep sadness and depression. You can imagine a hose that has pressure that can't come out or a person who eats and eats but does not release waste. Obviously they will eventually get sick – it's a question of time. It all stems from the imbalance of giving and receiving. Also a person who gives but doesn't receive is not in balance. This person might become drained. There is an explanation as to why the Dead Sea is so salty that nothing can live in its water, while the water in Sea of Galilee is sweet and has many fish living there. The reason is that while the Dead Sea only receives water from all the water sources around it; the Sea of Galilee receives and shares water to the point that it is the major source of water for the people in the area.

Generally speaking we are affected on 3 major levels: "guf" – the physical body, "nefesh" – food and environmental influences and "neshama" – the spiritual aspect i.e. what we read, see, hear and smell. The idea is to connect to Source in every facet of our life. Many times this way of thinking will help you to make the right choices in life.

When you don't know what kind of food to buy, think about how our food was initially created. Fruits and vegetables were not sprayed or genetically engineered. There was no processed and packaged food. Water didn't have chlorine added to it. Our clothes were not made from synthetic fabrics. Walls in houses did not have poisonous paint. The air didn't have car fumes and other pollutants. People got sunlight on a daily basis and exercise was a part of daily life. The list goes on. Each little thing is a little drop of light from the Ultimate Light. There are different worlds and layers where this system applies. It also applies in the nutritional world. If a person eats the wrong food, whatever comes out will reflect what they ate – it will have a bad odor and the person usually will not feel good after they have eaten. If this food doesn't come out of the body, it will begin to rot inside and this might lead to sickness.

On the other hand, if a person eats a lot of clean, healthy and nutritious food such as a lot of clean and fresh organic fruits and vegetables, the body will release waste in a much cleaner way. Many times the waste won't even have an odor. A person who eats this way may not even have any health issues. The person feels and looks better. They are glowing and their skin is glowing. It's all the same idea on different levels – spiritual, physical, etc. This food is Godliness; junk food is darkness. It's the opposite of Godliness. That's an example of how darkness can increase in the world.

 When you eat the wrong food, you usually get a stomach ache and you need to find a way to take this poison out of your system. Probably bad odors will be involved. When you're not doing what you need to do spiritually, you might get upset and angry and take it out on someone and unpleasant words may come out.

These forces i.e. light and dark are always fighting. If you light a match in a dark room, you have a little bit of light. Right away there is a force that is trying to put out the match. The match doesn't last and then you need another match. Imagine having a candle, a flashlight, electricity and finally daylight, the darkness will be pushed away. There is a constant war between light and darkness, impurity and Holiness.

It's all the same concept. The purer and more direct our connection with Source, the greater our ability to give this light in a cleaner, purer, holier and more effective way and then the light we add to the world will be stronger and more powerful. The idea is the same idea throughout, to be channel for light. To be a channel for Godliness, to receive Godliness and to give Godliness. The more people who will do it, the more Godliness and light there will be in the world. You receive light and you give light. When one person does it and then another person and so on, the light grows and grows, there is more and more light and less and less darkness, less and less impurity, fewer and fewer problems, fewer and fewer hardships; more health, less sickness; more light, less darkness; more "kedusha" (holiness), less impurity.

The idea is the same idea. The words are the same words. The names are slightly different. Each person uses names that they feel a connection to – it really doesn't matter. One of the ideas the Lubavitcher Rebbe talks about is the idea of "outreach". The whole idea of "Hassidut" (Hassidic teaching) and the vision of the Baal Shem Tov: you were lucky and Hashem gave you a certain light, give this light to others. Add more light to the world. If each person adds their light to the world, together we will drive darkness away from the world. Then truth will be revealed. If you know the truth, tell it to others. More truth, fewer lies and the closer we get to a world of truth and a state where all of us will be happier. That's also why it's important to tell the truth. It spreads light in the world.

We need to share our lights. We are all individuals and we all have special gifts – special light, a special candle and we are supposed to share our light, to pass a flame from candle to candle. That's the only way the puzzle will be complete and we'll reach illumination. Whatever good information and knowledge you merit to have, share it with as many people as possible. This way you will increase the light in the world to the maximum and will have room in your vessel to receive new light. The more light you give, the more light you receive and the greater levels of illumination you reach. On one hand it's a selfish concept but on a higher level, it's exactly the opposite. That's where many people get confused. We must keep the wheel going – receiving and giving, giving and receiving, etc. It's exactly this sense that a person will gain something from the experience that drives them to give to others.

We want to have the characteristics of the Creator as much as we can. Just like the Creator is kind, we need to be kind. Just like the Creator wants us to be healthy, we need to want other people to be healthy. Hashem wants to the world to be beautiful, so let's help each other to make the world beautiful. Just like Hashem talks to everyone, so too we need to speak the light to everyone and hope that their ears will be open. It's just a question of whether we are ready to hear and see the messages.

The "benefit" that Hashem "receives" is seeing His creation happy and illuminated. By the same token, our personal illumination will occur when we share our light with others and see the resulting illumination in others and in our entire planet. This is also the idea that all of us are each other's guarantors. The whole world is connected. Each person can add light and each person can add darkness – it's our choice. We are affected by each other and by our environment: our families, our neighbor, our city, our country and our planet. We can't run away from it. We are all in the same boat, actually the same planet. The closer you are to the true Godly teaching, the greater the light you can bring to the world and the greater your responsibility to do so. This applies to different levels – spiritually, nutritionally and physically. When will the optimal enlightenment be reached and when will the redemption arrive? When the wellsprings of Torah will be spread throughout the world, the light of Source will illuminate every corner of our planet and the world will be illuminated. It's not always easy to reach a perfect balance, especially when considering factors like making a living. This is the real struggle to find this point of balance. The minute you find this point of balance, you are illuminated. This is the true balance because Godliness is perfection. We need to strive to get there in a loving way. The more focused a person is, the less disturbances they have, the less sadness, the less anger, the less mood swings, because they are connected to Source. Connected to the Source of the soul connected to Hashem.

You might ask, "What about making a living?" The answer is that until the person reaches that point of balance – the right connection to Source, connecting to the rhythm of creation – they might need to look for a conventional way of earning a living. When we are connected to Source for the right reasons and in a balanced, clean and holy way in all aspects of our life – spiritually, physically and emotionally, our livelihood will find a way to reach us. Today, we are not part of the rhythm of the world. How do we connect to this rhythm – by doing what we need to on this planet. When we do what we need to in this world, then we reach full balance and it seems that everything happens on its own – that everything falls into place. It feels like a smooth ride on the "automatic pilot" of the universe. It's a Divine feeling.

Just like any machine that has one screw that is not connected properly, the whole machine cannot function. The moment the screw is connected, the machine works. Our job is to find our place, which screw we are. It might take time and energy but the moment we connect to the machine and the machine works smoothly and we experience the fruits of our efforts, we reach illumination and true happiness.

How do we know that we are on the right track? We have many tools. The first is to pay attention to our subconscious because we are aware of many things in our subconscious. Go within and ask ourselves questions, either out loud or to think of the question. "What do you think about this?" "Should I do this or should I do that?" You'll see that you receive answers. One of the ways to recognize if the answer is coming from the right place is if you hear an answer that is not exactly what you expected, but it's so accurate, pure and to the point, and the answer came suddenly and it sticks with you, it's usually your subconscious or the Godliness within you speaking. Another way to know is according to how we feel: when we feel a certain heaviness, anxiety or a need to run away, but on the other hand there are options which make us feel lighter, it might very well be that our psyche is hinting the right answer. It might take a little time to get the feel of how it works, but it's worth it, just to feel the connection to Source.

Sometimes we run away from our own truth or in other words from our connection to Source and we don't let the answer come freely. We need to nullify our preconceptions and put our thoughts and "brains" aside for a few minutes so the true answer will be able to come out. Another factor that might interfere with this process is that a person might, for whatever the reason, be running away from their purpose. Like in the story of Jonah, who was a prophet. He had a certain mission to fulfill and he tried to run away from it, but in the end, he had to face and fulfill his mission. If such a thing can happen to a prophet, who is on such an extreme spiritual level, it definitely can happen to each one of us. After all, each one of us has a mission to complete on our planet.

Feeling disturbed occurs when a person doesn't do what they have to do. When a person knows and does what they have to do, they are not disturbed. That's why you need to be busy with learning Divine concepts. This way you are constantly connected to Source and that's why you won't be disturbed, depressed, frustrated, etc. When you are connected to Source you can't go wrong because you are entirely connected to Godliness, the Source of your soul. When this happens, you are in perfect alignment and nothing can disturb you or disturb your thoughts and your entire being is channeling Godliness and this way there is "no entry" to negativity or unwanted thoughts.

After all, we are constantly busy with thinking and it's extremely hard to stop our thoughts. It's much easier and much more practical to keep ourselves busy with the right thoughts and make it a "no entry" for the rest. In other words, by keeping the light going, we're not letting the darkness in. When we let the darkness in, there is a danger it will overtake the light. It's the same concept in different versions and different words.

Someone who is constantly dealing with such teachings is constantly connected to Source and constantly connected to light. The stronger the connection to Source, the greater the light and the greater the potential for illumination. For this reason their soul will stay illuminated even when the body will disappear. This person will continue to live and will live even on a higher level because there won't be any physicality that will interfere with this illumination. That's why it says that true righteous people are greater in their death than in their life because the physicality doesn't interfere or take away from their spiritual light. As we know, the soul lives on forever.

One of the indications that a person is truly righteous and illuminated is when there is an unexplained desire to be next to them all the time. You feel a certain intangible sweetness and kindness that you can't explain. That's the Godliness and the light that we're all after. It's the rays of illumination. The minute we fit to the rhythm of the world and we do what we need to do spiritually, all the physical matters fall into place. We become part of the whole system. When you give what you need to give, you receive what you need. That can explain why sometimes we receive "gifts" out of nowhere.

Godliness is in everything. As mentioned in the introduction, the numerical value of one of the Hebrew Names of God is "Elokim". It's no coincidence that it has the same numerical value as the Hebrew word for nature "HaTeva". If you want to "know" the Creator, you need to know the creation. The Hebrew word for healthy is "bari", for creation is "briah" and for the Creator is "Boreh". These 3 words have the same 3 root letters. It's not a coincidence that in order to be "bari" - healthy, you need to strive to know and connect to the Creator - "Boreh" and that's done by knowing and connecting to His creation - "briah", which is our planet. That is why it's all one piece. If you want to reach illumination, you need to be connected to Source, you need to receive and give properly. If you want to know the Creator, get to know the creation, be connected to the creation, save the creation, respect the creation, keep the world clean, spiritually and physically, be passionate and loving towards the Creator, learn His teachings and be busy with His attributes, i.e. good deeds and kindness. In this way you will constantly be filled with Godliness. Then share this light with others. This is the concept of "baseless love", loving for the sake of loving and "baseless hatred", hating for no reason. This was the reason that Holy Temple in Jerusalem was destroyed. The Holy Temple was the House of Light. The destruction of the Temple reflects a lack of light. There was a lack of light because of "baseless hatred" which is manifested when people don't give to each other, when there is a lack of "baseless love". When there is "baseless love" we have the Holy Temple. The Holy Temple exists when we give and when we give there is Godliness in the world. It is all connected.

The point is "baseless love" and "baseless hatred". There is Godliness in the world, when you give Godliness to others, if you learned something, give it to others, teach others. This is "baseless love". In this way our Holy Temple will be rebuilt, the darkness will disappear from the world. The destruction is "baseless hatred", when a person doesn't give their wisdom to others. We see another example with the students of Rabbi Akiva. They didn't respect each other and as a result, 24,000 students died in a plague – there was darkness. Try to imagine 24,000 students like Rabbi Meir and Rabbi Shimon bar Yochai how much light could have been in the world. What was the teaching of Rabbi Akiva, who was their rabbi? "Veahavta lereaacha kamocha" (love your neighbor as yourself) or "baseless love". That is the medicine and the entire Godly teaching in brief. By giving to others we merit to constantly be connected to the true and Infinite Light. Learn, teach and do.

The same concept is repeated in many places as the Rebbe explains in the discourse "Lecha Dodi" that it's all about giving and receiving. Just like the six days of the week give to the seventh and the seventh gives to the other six. The six attributes "zeir anpin" (the six days of the week) and kingship "malchut" (the seventh day) are like a husband and a wife. If the giving and receiving between a husband and wife is done properly, the woman who begins as "malchut" becomes the crown of her husband "keter" and "keter" is an extremely high level of light as explained according to kabbalah and hassidut.

It's explained that the blood affects the soul "...for the blood is the soul ("nefesh")..." (Deuteronomy 12:23). So whoever cares about his soul should care about what is nourishing his body. In other words, "you are what you eat".

The less darkness, the more light and truth will be revealed in the world. We'll be able to open our eyes and understand the toxins in our planet and our society that we are surrounded by without being aware of it, like the food we eat, the water we drink and the air we breathe. The more truth will be spread in the world, the faster the darkness will disappear. When this happens, we'll all be happier and we'll be able to see Godliness with our own eyes. We all can and should do it – we all deserve it...."Since, this thing is very close to you; it is in your mouth and in your heart, to do it" (Deuteronomy 30:14).

There are many different ways to connect to Source - learning Divine concepts ("talmud Torah"), talking to Source ("tefillah") and doing good deeds ("gemilut hasadim"). Whatever we do to connect, we should do with our thought, speech and action. The better and more accurately we do it, the closer we get to our place we need to be in the universe. Doing good deeds ("mitzvot" and "gemilut hasadim") is especially important because these are illumination on a physical level. "Lishma" (for no personal benefit) is when people learn Torah so that they will be able to do whatever they need to on this planet. Being connected to Source is in everything we do: health, healing, sport and nutrition. The more we connect to Source and nature, the way things were meant to be in their natural state, the closer we will get to where we need to be in God's plan, our purpose. The more we do this, the more we will feel the light, flow and abundance from Above.

Whoever merits receiving the Godly Light has an even greater task to spread this light in the world. He who receives the light has the job to be this light, to be a light to all others, to give a good example. Perhaps that's why the expectations from such a person are greater. As soon as a person merits succeeding in this task they have the potential to reach great illumination. The minute a person reaches this state they can understand and appreciate the merit they have and how blessed they are.

32

The Sum of the Matter

After this life, or as some call it, "In the world to come, (the world of souls) there is no body or physical form, only the souls alone, without a body, like the ministering angels. Since there is no physical form, there is neither eating, drinking, nor any of the other bodily functions of this world like sitting, standing, sleeping, death, sadness, laughter, and the like...but the righteous will sit with their crowns on their heads and delight in the radiance of the Divine Presence.

They will have the knowledge that they achieved, which allowed them to merit the life of the world to come. This will be their crown. As King Solomon says: "The crown with which his mother crowned him" (Song of Songs 3:11). "Eternal joy will be upon their heads" (Isaiah 51:11). They will comprehend the truth of Godliness which they cannot grasp while in a body (Rambam Teshuva 8:2). This is hinted in King David's statement: "How great is the good that You have hidden for those who respect You" (Psalms 31:20).

"One who serves out of love occupies himself in the Torah and good deeds "mitzvot" and walks in the paths of wisdom for no ulterior motive: not because of fear that evil will occur, nor in order to acquire benefit. Rather, he does what is true because it is true, and ultimately, good will come because of it…" (Rambam Teshuvah 10:2). As it says, "you should love Hashem your God with all your heart and all your soul and with all you have" (Deuteronomy 6:5).

Rabbi Shimlai said 613 commandments were told to Moses on Mount Sinai, 365 negative commandments as the number of the days of the sun and 248 positives commandments parallel to the number of the organs of man. Came David and put them into eleven: "A psalm by David. Hashem who may abide in Your tent? Who may dwell on Your holy Mountain? He who walks in perfect innocence, acts justly, and speaks truth in his heart; who has no slander on his tongue, who has done his fellowman no evil, and who has brought no disgrace upon his relative; in whose eyes a despicable person is repulsive, but who honors those who are

God-fearing; who does not change his oath even if it is to his own detriment; who does not lend his money at interest, nor accept a bribe against the innocent. He who does these things shall not falter forever" (Psalm 15). Came Isaiah and put them into six: "Which of us can live with the Eternal Fire? One who walks with righteousness and speaks with truthfulness, who is repulsed by extortion and shakes off his hands from holding a bribe, who seals his ears from hearing of bloodshed and shuts his eyes from seeing bad. He will dwell in heights; in rocky fortresses is his stronghold. His bread will be granted, his water assured" (Isaiah 33:14-16). Came Micah and put them into three: "With what will I approach Hashem, humble myself before God on high?...He has told you, o man what is good, what does Hashem require of you but to do justice, to love kindness and to walk humbly with your God (Micah 6:6, 8).

Came again Isaiah and put them into two: "So said Hashem: Observe justice and perform righteousness for My salvation is soon to come and My righteousness to be revealed" (Isaiah 56:1). Came Amos and put them into one: "So said Hashem to the House of Israel: Seek Me and live (Amos 5:4). Came Havakuk and put them into one: "...a righteous person through his faith will live" (Havakuk 2:4) (Talmud Makot 23 p. 2). "Who may ascend the mountain of Hashem, and who may stand in His holy place? He who has clean hands and a pure heart, who has not used My Name in vain or sworn falsely. He shall receive a blessing from Hashem, and kindness from God, his deliverer" (Psalms 24:3-5). "There are six things that Hashem deeply dislikes and the seventh is an abomination of His soul; haughty eyes, a lying tongue, and hands that shed innocent blood; a heart that thinks thoughts of violence; feet that hasten to run to bad; speaks lies with false testimony and incites quarrels among brothers" (Proverbs 6:16-19).

"A certain heathen came before Hillel and said to him, "Make me a convert, on the condition that you teach me the whole Torah while I stand on one foot." Hillel replied, "What is hateful to you, do not do to your neighbor: that is the whole Torah while the rest is commentary; go and learn it" (Talmud Shabbat 31a). Rabbi Akiva says: "…Love your fellow as you love yourself…"(Leviticus 19:18), and he added "it's a fundamental rule in the Torah" (Talmud Yerushalmi Nedarim 9).

"The sum of the matter, when all has been considered: Have awe towards your Creator and keep His commandments, for that is a man's whole duty" (Ecclesiastes 12:13).

Learn wisdom, keep your thoughts positive, keep your speech to a minimum, eat as little and as wholesome as you can, dwell in a healthy environment, love and appreciate the Creator and the creations: the environment, plants, animals and each other, surround yourself with people you love and trust and practice giving and receiving kindness and love.

33

25 Days of Contemplation

DAY 1

Being Thankful.

Be thankful for the things you have.

Remember you have a lot to be thankful for.

DAY 2

Family and Friends.

Spend more time with family and friends.

Try to be surrounded by people who make you feel good.

Treat yourself to more quality time. Start by leaving the television and computer off.

DAY 3

Sense Therapy.

Remember that everything you see, hear, speak, eat,

breathe, think and experience has an effect on you.

DAY 4
What we see.

Pay attention to what you see throughout the day: what you read, watch on TV or view on the computer.

We tend to think that only our children need to be protected from what they see.

Positive media will have a positive effect on your life.

DAY 5
What we hear.

Everything you hear has an effect on you.

Stay away from gossip and empty conversations.

Switch off unnecessary noise sources such as the radio, television, humming computer, etc.

A quiet environment is a calming environment.

DAY 6
What we say.

Using positive words and expressions will have an enormous effect on how you feel and your interactions with others.

Imagine that every word spoken is a dollar out of your pocket – think twice about what you say.

Saving words means saving energy.

DAY 7
What we eat.

Visit your fridge and pantry:
Get rid of all the junk food- anything with hydroge-
nated oils, trans fats, refined sugar and soft drinks.
Read food labels.

DAY 8
What we should eat.
Eat a balanced preferably organic and live diet rich in
fresh fruits and vegetables adding some whole grains,
nuts and seeds, as packed as possible with enzymes. (If
you can't get organic try to peel or wash with natural
soap.)
Drink enough clean water; many say 8 glasses a day is
a good place to start. Try to keep away from soft
drinks, caffeine, hydrogenated oils, processed food and
refined sugars.

DAY 9
What we breathe.
Clean air is one of the foundations of life.
Look for a location that is known for its air quality. Try
to be surrounded by trees and greenery.
Make sure to air your house with fresh air every day.
Green plants are a wonderful way to purify the air in
your home or office.

DAY 10
What we think.
Recognize and push negative thoughts out of your

head.

Positive thinking is healing and helpful in preventing sickness and premature aging.

Closing your eyes for a few minutes and imagining yourself in a positive and healing place can lower your stress levels.

Thinking is a very powerful tool.

DAY 11

Character Therapy.

Stay away from sadness, anger, jealousy, pride, and so on.

Such traits originate from not being able to see the whole picture.

Believing that everything happens for good, is a great way to start overcoming these.

DAY 12

Money management.

Make a table of your monthly income, expenses, debts, loans, etc.

Prioritize your expenses and see if there is anything that can be taken off the list.

Try to balance your budget so that you can cover all your expenses and still have some money to put aside.

It's all about how much we save, not how much we make.

DAY 13
Time Management.
Make a weekly "To Do List" – remember to include time to eat, sleep, etc.
Break it up into daily tasks.
Organize each day realistically – don't overload it.
Time is very precious. Try to make the most of it.

DAY 14
Do a good deed.
Put aside time to volunteer and help others.
You'll be surprised how much you'll grow from it.

DAY 15
Keep yourself in check.
Routine checkups at your dentist and family doctor are really important for peace of mind. Remember to ask for complete blood work and an EKG test. Don't forget to check for vitamin D and B12. A deficiency can easily be solved with supplements.
It might also save you money in the long run.

DAY 16
Stretches.
Stretching for a few minutes a day on a regular basis is extremely beneficial.
It can improve blood flow, bodily function and greatly enhance your mood.
Basic stretches such as touching your toes, reaching to

the side and reaching to the ceiling are a great way to start.

DAY 17
Exercise.
Moderate exercise such as taking a brisk walk for 30 minutes a day, 5 times a week can greatly improve your general mood and overall fitness.
Choose an area with fresh, clean air and trees.
Air tends to be cleaner first thing in the morning and as far away from traffic as possible.

DAY 18
Water Therapy.
Take a bath or shower everyday and change into clean clothes.
It's a great, simple way to feel refreshed and relaxed.
Many people find it helpful to do an enema once a month.

DAY 19
Sleep Therapy.
Get around 8 hours of sleep a night.
Go to bed early and try to get up before sunrise.
Getting enough quality sleep is very therapeutic and has a healing effect on your body.

DAY 20
Light and Color.

Open the blinds and let direct sunlight in.

Pay attention to lighting, soft light tends to improve your general mood.

Choose the colors around you such as furniture and wall color and surround yourself with colors that make you feel good.

DAY 21

Color Therapy Tips.

Blue: Relaxation, truth.

Purple: Spirituality, peacefulness.

Red: Stimulation, passion, energy.

Orange: Optimism.

Yellow: Mental ability, awakening.

Green: Growth, healing, calming.

Pink: Soothing.

Grey: Safe, comforting.

Brown: Grounding.

White: Purity, truth, innocence.

Black: Power.

DAY 22

Divine Design Tips.

Keep the front door area free of objects.

Avoid clutter. Place things where they belong.

Take care of unpleasant odors, using natural, fragrances only. Natural, scented oils are a great idea.

Place a water feature in your house.

Avoid having a T.V. and or mirrors in your bedroom.

Make sure that your mattress has a solid wall behind it and is resting on legs. Allow air to pass under it.

DAY 23
Music Therapy.
Treat yourself to a relaxing CD.
Set aside time to lay down comfortably.
Listen and focus on the music, while practicing deep breathing.
Listening to relaxing music is like yoga for the mind.

DAY 24
Nature Therapy.
Find a green, peaceful corner with fresh, clean air.
Clear your mind and thoughts by having your lunch there or just spending some quiet down time.
Try to get some sunlight.
Your local park can be a great place to begin.

DAY 25
Schedule a vacation.
When was the last time you got away and had some good and relaxing quality time?
It doesn't have to be far away nor expensive.

34

Self Coaching

DAY 1
Admit your feelings and accept them.
Identify sources of stress and try to eliminate them.

DAY 2
Find a peaceful place, where you can actually hear yourself think.
It can be your backyard, your porch, a park, whatever works for you.
It's a great place to be thankful for what you have and to ask for what you wish to have.
This peaceful place is the beginning of your journey.

DAY 3
Live Coaching, involves making decisions through

speaking and listening to a coach in their office.

Self Coaching involves making decisions through reading and writing in your journal. The location is up to you.

DAY 4

Self Coaching is great because you can write whenever and wherever you want.

You can also go back and read through what you wrote. No need to "choose" your words or think twice about revealing your secrets.

DAY 5

Try to write in a journal every day. This is very important, since your journal will act as your Coach.

By looking through your journal after a while, you will begin to see patterns in your life. This will make it easier for you to select your goals and work towards them.

DAY 6

Make a list in your journal.

Write down the things in your life that you always wanted to change or improve.

Prioritize your list.

Make sure your goals are realistic.

DAY 7

Choose a goal and break it into:

Truth: Where are you now?

Goals: Where would you like to be?
Tools: What actions can you take to get there?
Obstacles: What things do you feel might stop you?
Solutions: How can you overcome them?
Time: In what time frame would you like to get there?

DAY 8
Example:
Truth: I'm overweight.
Goals: I'd like to lose 10 lb.
Tools: Exercise, go on diet, not to eat late at night.
Obstacles: Cravings and cold weather (harder to exercise).
Solutions: Have healthy snacks handy for cravings. Power walk in the mall.
Time: Within 3 months.

DAY 9
Re-evaluate your goal at the end of the time frame. It's okay if you are no longer interested in it or need to rethink your ways to get there.
It's part of learning about yourself and finding out what you really want.
Put closure on one goal before moving onto the next.
Remember big steps are made of small steps.

DAY 10
Smile.
Remember deep breathing and laughing.

Try to tell or hear a joke once a day.
Don't take life too seriously.
Happiness is a state of mind, not a state of location.

AN IDEA FOR A DAILY SCHEDULE

Psalms

Stretching

2 liters water

Green leaf based strained juice

Big live veggie salad

Fruit smoothie – not juice! (apples, bananas, pears)

Soup or zucchini pasta

Exercise: cardio like walking, jogging, cycling, basketball, etc.

Shower – scrub with loofah

Floss and brush teeth and tongue twice a day

Early to bed, at least 8 hours of sleep

35

RECIPES

1. VEGAN GREEK SALAD

Ingredients
150 g firm tofu
3 medium sized cucumbers
2 tomatoes
3 romaine lettuce leaves
½ cup black olives
¼ cup fresh lemon juice
1 tablespoon olive oil (optional)
½ teaspoon salt (optional)
1 small red onion (optional)

Preparation
Grate the tofu and place in a small bowl. Pour half the lemon juice onto the grated tofu. Add half the sea salt (optional).

Chop the cucumbers, tomatoes, lettuce and onion.
Place in a large bowl.
Add the lemon juice and olive oil to the vegetables.
Mix gently.
Sprinkle the tofu and olives on top.
Serve and enjoy!

2. GLUTEN FREE TABOULI SALAD

Ingredients
1 small cauliflower
2 cucumbers
1 tomato
¼ cup fresh parsley
¼ to ½ cup fresh lemon juice
1 teaspoon olive oil
Sea salt (optional)

Preparation
Finley chop the cauliflower in a food processor using
the "s" blade. Place in a large bowl.
Cut the cucumbers and tomato into small cubes. Add
to the chopped cauliflower.
Finely chop the parsley. Add to the vegetables.
Add the lemon juice, olive oil and sea salt to taste.
Mix, serve and enjoy!

3. BEET & TAHINI SALAD

Ingredients
2 beets
¼ cup lemon juice
¼ cup chopped onion
¼ cup tahini sauce

Preparation
Grate beets.
Mix in lemon juice, onion and tahini sauce.
Serve and enjoy!

4. CABBAGE & DILL SALAD

Ingredients
1 small cabbage
½ bunch of fresh dill
¼ cup lemon juice
2 tablespoons of olive oil
¼ teaspoon of sea salt

Preparation
Shred the cabbage.
Massage in sea salt to soften the cabbage.
Chop the dill and add to the cabbage.
Add the lemon juice and olive oil.
Mix, serve and enjoy!

5. VEGAN CHEESE PASTA

Ingredients
3 large and long zucchinis
½ cup fresh lemon juice
1 cup sesame paste (tahini sauce)
¼ cup of water
¼ teaspoon oregano
sea salt to taste (optional)
¼ cup of sundried tomatoes (optional)

Preparation
Make the pasta using a vegetable spiralizer (a must!)

Blend the remaining ingredients in a blender. Pour over the pasta. (Feel free to add more or less water to achieve the
desired consistency.)
Serve and enjoy!

Cheese Variation:
2 cups of raw cashews soaked overnight and rinsed
¼ cup of nutritional yeast

6. HEALTHY KETCHUP

Ingredients
1 cup sundried tomatoes soaked in 2 teaspoons of olive oil
1 ½ cups fresh tomatoes
3-6 teaspoons apple cider vinegar
2 dates
1 teaspoon paprika
1 teaspoon onion powder
½ teaspoon of sea salt

Preparation
Blend and enjoy!

7. HEALTHY VEGAN MAYONNAISE

Ingredients
2 tablespoons of raw cashews
2 cups of coconut meat
½ to 1 cup of apple cider vinegar
¾ cup of olive oil
½ cup of water
2 teaspoons of sea salt

Preparation
Blend and enjoy!

8. APPLE OR GRAPE SLUSH

Ingredients
3 pounds (1.5 kg) grapes or 10 sweet apples

Preparation
Separate grapes from the stems or core the apples.
Wash and rinse well.
Blend in a blender.
Freeze.
Partially defrost and enjoy – great for kids!

9. DATE BANANA SMOOTHIE

Ingredients
5 ripe spotted bananas (partially frozen).
10 pitted dates.
A handful of nuts or almonds (soaked and rinsed).
Clean and pure water to cover the fruit.

Preparation
Blend in a blender and enjoy!

10. PEANUT BUTTER BANANA SMOOTHIE

Ingredients
5 ripe spotted bananas (partially frozen)
10 pitted dates
2 heaped tablespoons organic peanut butter
Clean and pure water to cover the fruit

Preparation
Blend in a blender and enjoy!

11. FIG BANANA SMOOTHIE

Ingredients
5 ripe spotted bananas (partially frozen)
15 dried figs
Clean and pure water to cover the fruit

Preparation
Blend in a blender and enjoy!

12. VEGAN CHOCOLATE MILK

Ingredients
200 g pitted dates
1-2 teaspoons of sesame butter
1-2 tablespoons of carob powder
3-4 8 oz cups of water (cold or warm)

Preparation
Place all the ingredients in a blender.
Blend until smooth and enjoy!

13. VEGAN PIE CRUST

Ingredients
400 g pitted dates or dried figs
100 g crushed nuts
½ teaspoon ginger (optional)
½ teaspoon cinnamon (optional)

Preparation
Place the dates in the food processor. Using the "s" blade mix until combined into a ball.
Put the dates and the remaining ingredients into a bowl. Squish by hand until combined.
Lay it flat on the base of a spring-form pan – this is your crust that you can use as a base for any "cake".

14. VEGAN APPLE PIE

Ingredients
Pie Crust (Please see recipe.)
8 apples (the sweeter the better).
½ teaspoon cinnamon
½ cup raisins (optional)

Preparation
Chop apples in the food processor using the "s" blade.
Mix in the cinnamon and raisins.
Spread over the crust.
Decorate using apple slices, nuts and or dates. Be creative and have fun!
Serve at room temperature or chilled to taste and enjoy!

15. VEGAN BANANA PIE

Ingredients
Pie Crust (Please see recipe.)
10 spotted ripe bananas
½ teaspoon cinnamon
½ cup raisins (optional)

Preparation
Mash the bananas using a fork.
Mix in the cinnamon and raisins.
Spread over the crust.
Decorate using banana slices, nuts and or dates.
Serve at room temperature or chilled to taste and
enjoy!

16. VEGAN BANANA HALVA PIE

Ingredients
Pie Crust (Please see recipe.)
10 spotted ripe bananas
½ teaspoon cinnamon
1 cup of crushed halva (without hydrogenated oils)

Preparation
Mash the bananas using a fork.
Mix in the cinnamon.
Spread half of the banana filling over the crust.
Sprinkle half of the crushed halva over the banana
filling.
Spoon the other half of the banana filling over the
halva.
Sprinkle the remaining halva over the banana filling.
Decorate using banana slices, nuts and or dates.
Serve at room temperature or chilled to taste and
enjoy!

17. VEGAN MANGO BANANA PIE

Ingredients
Pie Crust (Please see recipe.)
7 spotted ripe bananas

2 large ripe mangos

Preparation
Mash the bananas using a fork.
Mash the mangos.
Spread half of the crushed bananas over the crust.
Spread half of the crushed mangos over the crust.
Spread the other half of the crushed bananas over the mangos.
Spread the other half of the crushed mangos over the bananas.
Decorate using banana slices, nuts and or dates.
Serve at room temperature or chilled to taste and enjoy!

18. VEGAN CHOCOLATE BALLS

Ingredients
400 g pitted dates or dried figs
100 g crushed nuts
1 tablespoon of carob powder
Stone-ground almond butter (optional)

Preparation
Place the dates and carob powder in the food processor. Using the "s" blade mix until combined into a ball.
Put the dates and nuts into a bowl. Squish by hand until combined.
Form into small balls.
(For an extra kick dip each ball into almond butter.)
Serve at room temperature or chilled to taste and enjoy!

19. VEGAN BROWNIES

Ingredients
400 g pitted dates or dried figs
100 g crushed nuts
1-2 tablespoons of carob powder

Preparation
Place the dates and carob powder in the food processor. Using the "s" blade mix until combined into a ball.
Put the dates and nuts into a bowl. Squish by hand until combined.
Spread and press into a tray at least an inch thick.
Cut into squares.
Serve at room temperature or chilled to taste and enjoy!

20. DATE TRUFFLES

Ingredients
Pitted dates
Sesame butter

Preparation
Open each date while still attached on one side.
Place some sesame butter on one half and "close" the date.
Enjoy!

ABOUT THE AUTHOR

After traveling the Unites States, Australia, Europe and Far East Asia for several years, Oren received his degree in respiratory therapy while living in Colorado. He felt like his searching had just started. The monk's words from the monastery, "Go back to your religion you have everything you need there." kept echoing in his head and he decided to continue to religious studies and ordination. While caring for his parents, he realized the fundamental need for knowledge in natural healing and environmental awareness and decided to pursue a degree in holistic and sports nutrition. Oren is the author of the popular three-volume children's series "Super Danny".

...he planted an Oren tree, and rain makes it grow...   Isaiah 44:14

To you the reader and to my dearest Leah and Gabriel.

DISCLAIMER

This book is not coming to serve as medical advice or to teach "halacha". Any decisions and actions taken are the full responsibility of the reader.

www.ingramcontent.com/pod-product-compliance
Lightning Source LLC
Chambersburg PA
CBHW051252250726
48656CB00004B/1255